Contents

Acknowledgements

The work reported here stems from a research project in the South West of England. We are very grateful to our funders, the NHS Executive South and West, who generously supported the work.

This report deals with the issues arising from the main part of the project, during which we interviewed families who had just received an assessment. It would not have been possible without the cooperation of the five social services departments that took part in the study, and in particular, the professional teams and day services staff who were carrying out assessments, and allowed us to examine their practice. We are very grateful to all these people.

We would also like to thank all the members of our research advisory group, who have read through drafts of this report and helped us to represent fairly a range of perspectives:

Robina Mallett (carer/carers' officer with Home Farm Trust)

Penny Banks (King's Fund Centre)

Emily Holzhausen (Carers' National Association)

David Myatt (Devon Social Services)

Claire Gazdar (Department of Health)

Neil Palmer (self-advocate and representative of the project focus group)

Bryony Beresford (researcher)

We have also had a focus group of self-advocates who have given us advice, and we would like to say thank you to:

Neil Palmer

Tiffany England

Tracy Fry

Matthew Whyte

We are also grateful to the many groups of carers and individuals who helped by telling us what their main concerns were. One group deserves a special mention, the South East Bristol Carers' Group. They have always provided a warm welcome and checked through the questions we planned to ask in our interviews with carers.

We were fortunate to have the support of Harry Wishart and Debbie Watson, who helped with the interviewing, and Carol Eddon and Jennifer Stirratt, who did some of the transcription work. Karen Gyde, from the Norah Fry Research Centre, has provided invaluable secretarial support and we are most grateful for her conscientious work. Finally, Pat Simmons did a stalwart job on proof reading and editing the final version.

Last but not least, of course, we would like to thank all the 51 carers and the people with learning disabilities, who gave up their time to talk so frankly with us about their own needs and experiences. Without their words, their insight, and their commitment, this report could not have been written.

Notes about terminology

- The term 'carer's needs assessment' has been used throughout, since carers in this study told us that 'carer assessment' had negative associations for them, and made them feel as though they were being put to the test. We felt that 'carer's needs assessment' is a more accurate description.

- Service reviews are usually referred to as 'IPP', which stands for Individual Programme Plan. In some of the areas in which we worked the service review was called IP or ISP, but we will generally use the acronym IPP in this report.

- This report uses the terminology 'people with learning difficulties' in accordance with Department of Heath practice, since the research project was funded by the NHS Executive.

- Carers can be male or female, and so we have alternated references to he/she and him/her in the text.

Executive summary

Aim

The aim of this research project was to find out whether the Carers Act was working for carers of people with learning disabilities. The Carers Act gave those providing 'regular and substantial care' the right to an assessment of their own needs.

Methods

We worked in five local authorities in the South West of England. Two of these were mainly rural areas, the others were urban. We carried out:

- a records search to discover the proportion of eligible carers receiving a carer's needs assessment over a year;
- interviews with 51 carers of people with learning disabilities who either had been assessed under the Carers Act or had had their needs taken into account at a service review;
- interviews or meetings with the people with learning disabilities involved;
- a further examination of assessment records;
- follow-up interviews approximately one year later with the carers.

All interviews were analysed qualitatively whereas the records data were analysed quantitatively.

Findings

- Over a quarter of carers in this study had chronic health problems or impairments and over a third were caring for another disabled person apart from the person with learning disabilities.

- Across the five areas, of 157 eligible carers, only 22% had received a full carer's needs assessment between April 1997 and March 1998. A further 50% had had their needs taken into account to some extent and there was some evidence of this on care plans, but 28% had not had their needs assessed at all.

- Those people with learning disabilities who had a community care or Children Act assessment tended to be in crisis or at a major transition point. For most carers, the legal triggers to a Carers Act assessment were therefore not likely to happen. The best they could hope for was some recognition of their needs at the service review (usually an IPP or similar) but this is usually very focused on the service user.

- An analysis of the full and partial assessments that did take place indicates that some key aspects of carers' lives were often not discussed, including their health, housing, work and ability to continue caring.

- Publicity about the Carers Act did not seem to have reached most carers we met. Only one had requested an assessment as a direct result of a publicity leaflet.

- Record keeping was found to be poor and sometimes did not provide a good account of the needs, the decisions or the plans for the future. Assessment forms were sometimes disliked by professionals and needed to be amended to make them more flexible.

- People with learning disabilities were generally accepting of their carers' needs and some understood their need for support and short breaks from them.

- Some people with learning disabilities were starting to take on caring tasks for elderly parents, and families were becoming mutually dependent.
- Carers told us their greatest concern was the future care of their relative and many seemed to lack information about what might be possible.
- Carers found their assessments most useful when they felt their needs and those of their relative were considered carefully and privately. Advocates were important for both carers and people with learning disabilities.
- Carers tended to view their needs as inseparable from those of their relative and argued that if community support for the person with learning disabilities was good, they would have no needs.
- Many carers were fearful about planned changes to services, particularly day care. This is not surprising when some had had bad experiences of promises for services not being kept.
- Outcomes of carers' needs assessments were very poor. Only 18 of the 42 services that had been discussed in the carer's needs assessments had been provided after approximately one year.

Recommendations

At present the majority of carers of people with learning disabilities do *not* get a carer's needs assessment. Therefore our report recommends that local authorities should take a fresh look at the support they give to carers of people with learning disabilities, and consider some of the following.

Carer support workers

Carer support workers were regarded by carers as independent and 'on the carer's side'.

More carer support workers should be employed, and in some cases they should be enabled to carry out the carer assessment, provided that their role is understood by all, and that their authority to identify needs and suggest resources is respected by budget holders.

Day services

If **day services** are expected to help families plan for the future and access services, authorities should consider some of the following:

- a designated role of carer support officer within each day centre or day service, who could ensure that all staff know of their responsibility to involve, inform and support carers;
- a policy of seeing all carers personally in their own home, if possible, for a discussion that would be similar to a carer's needs assessment, perhaps at the time of the IPP (service review) meeting;
- staff training (perhaps provided by carers) in carer issues;
- an information and advice service within day centres or other forms of day service.

People with a learning disabiity

People with a learning disability should have:

- a designated keyworker, acting in many respects as an advocate;
- a right to a one:one discussion prior to their IPP meeting;
- staff who are trained in disability rights issues;
- accessible information and communication strategies.

Support to people with learning disabilities who become carers

Social services departments should work out a strategy to give information, support and access to carer assessments to people with learning disabilities who are becoming carers themselves. They need:

- an assessment of their needs as carers;
- formal support;
- appropriate training.

More research and development should be carried out into this issue.

Round table discussions

In addition to separate private meetings for the carer and the individual with learning disabilities, there should be provision for a round table discussion with the individual, the carer and all the professionals involved.

Staff training

- Clarify for all relevant staff who is entitled to a carer's needs assessment, and how they intend to deliver this commitment.

- Ensure that all relevant staff, including those who work with disabled children, understand the purpose of the carer's needs assessment and what it implies.

- Involve carers of people with learning disabilities in staff training.

- Involve people with learning disabilities (self-advocates) in staff training about disability equality issues.

- Ensure that the person delivering a carer's needs assessment can make clear to the carer the purpose and import of what is happening.

- Plan a strategy to enable people with learning disabilities themselves to access carer's needs assessments, when they start to take on caring roles.

Information

Authorities should develop and regularly monitor a strategy for providing information to carers of people with learning disabilities, including:

- information points at day centres and other day services, for carers as well as for people with learning disabilities;

- newsletters distributed directly to families;

- leaflets;

- talks and discussion at carer centres and carer groups.

Social services departments need to have a clear policy about carers' needs assessments and give better information to carers about them.

Records

Local authorities should review their record keeping systems for carer's needs assessments, taking into account the following factors:

- records should be seen as an aid to the carer's needs assessment process;

- forms for recording carers' needs should be developed in conjunction with representative groups of carers, as some authorities have already done;

- records should be concise and clear: they should be readable for carers and families, and also produced in an accessible format, so that the people with learning disabilities can understand their own assessment;

- records should be quick to complete, and preferably in a uniform format so that everyone (families and assessors) understands records when they move from one system to another, for example from children's to adults' services;

- records should be available to all parties concerned, especially the carer and the person with learning disabilities.

Future planning

There should be a coordinated and continuous service response to the family, that:

- includes both the carer and the person with learning disabilities;

- gives clear, concrete information about life-styles and future options, for example by direct visits to residential options, employment and leisure pursuits, and by written information, access to newsletters and data banks;

- provides the family with role models for the future, for example by meeting people with learning disabilities, including self-advocates, who are living more independently;

- gives a positive and clear message that the person with learning disabilities has rights to appropriate support outside the family situation;

- records the wishes of both the carer and the individual, at regular intervals, so that a life plan is gradually developed, that can be built on and altered as circumstances change.

It is important that future planning is stressed in the government's agenda on carers.

Carers themselves recognised that the key for good carer support is to provide good community support for people with learning disabilities. Local authorities must not see carer support as a substitute for improvements in services for people with learning disabilities.

Introduction

Background

In their own right was a research project about the implementation of the Carers Act of 1995. Unlike many other projects concerning carers, this was specifically about families with a member who had been defined as having a learning disability. Many of the issues for the carer are the same in these families as in other caring situations (see, for example, Twigg and Atkin, 1994), but there are also significant differences. Carers of people with learning disabilities often experience what Todd and Shearn (1996) describe as "perpetual parenthood" (p 393).

Two years after the implementation of the Carers Act, our aim was to look in depth at the experience of carer's needs assessments, and how they were carried out. We wanted to find out what the carer and the disabled person felt about assessments, and how their perceptions compared with that of the local authority and with each other's.

It is now well recognised that carers are not always aware that they have had, or been offered, an assessment (DoH, 1995; Holzhausen, 1997). In addition, others have highlighted the negative aspects of assessments. For example, Dobson (1995) referred to potential fears and insecurity associated with an assessment.

> *What it feels like to have people coming into your home, looking into your business, and then disappearing.* (p 10)

The Carers National Association (CNA) surveys (1995) showed that the satisfaction level of carers with their own assessments dropped between 1993 and 1994. Only 40% considered their own needs met, and in 1997, one year after the implementation of the Carers Act, Holzhausen (1997) found that the situation had still not significantly improved.

Therefore there are many good reasons to focus on the assessment process. Since we interviewed carers shortly after their carer's needs assessments, we were able to point out both the shortcomings from their perspective, and also the good practice. We aimed for a constructive approach.

Carers and those they care for: a shared agenda?

Writers who adopt a social model of disability, in particular those who are disabled themselves, have provided a strong critique of the Carers Movement (see Morris, 1993, 1994) for not taking into account the desire of disabled people to be in control of their own support. The very terminology of 'carer' and 'cared for' emphasises the dependency of the disabled person, and the literature on caring has often painted a negative picture of disabled people as 'a burden'. A focus on carers' needs can obscure:

> *... the social and economic inequalities which lie at the heart of those difficulties (the difficulties imposed on disabled people by society).* (Morris, 1993, p 33)

Similarly, Parker (1994) highlights the conflict between the individual disabled person's need for autonomy, and the interests of parents, family and society at large.

Some recent writers, however, have urged us to be aware of the 'shared agenda' between carer and disabled person. Twigg and Atkin (1994) and Todd and Shearn (1996) suggest an approach which takes into account the relationship and the common interests of both parties:

> *... developing an agenda of shared issues ... rather than the more usual situation where the difficulties one party encounters tend to be attributed to the other.* (Todd and Shearn, 1996, p 398)

Nolan et al (1996) also look to mutuality of care as a source of satisfaction for carers, and Grant and

Whittell (1999) found that a positive attitude in the 'cared for' person could be a major reward for the carer.

In the area of learning disability services, despite the legal rights now enjoyed by disabled people themselves, for instance under the 1990 NHS and Community Care Act, the carer has always had a strong voice in terms of articulating needs and advocating in the best interests of the disabled person, who in some cases literally cannot speak for him/herself (see Beresford, 1995; Walmsley, 1996). It is hard for parents to move beyond the 'parental role' (see Richardson and Ritchie, 1989; Todd and Shearn, 1996); these carers are people who may well have taken on a life-long commitment to caring. With someone with a learning disability, 'caring' can be synonymous with 'being responsible for' and this creates a relationship that has to be handled very sensitively in order to avoid tensions.

This study follows the work of Walmsley (1993, 1996) which recognises that the caring situation is a complex one involving at least two people within the family, who will occasionally be taking reciprocal caring roles, and who both have needs, views and rights. Walmsley (1996) noted that research into the 'caring' relationship has focused exclusively on the carer's perspective. Family carers have been enabled to construct their own identities, and have been instrumental in their presentation of themselves and of family life (Richardson and Ritchie, 1989; Grant and Nolan, 1993; Shearn and Todd, 1997).

The recent NHS Executive report *Signposts for success ...* (1998) noted that:

> *A distinction should be made between the views of service users and carers – these are not necessarily the same and this can lead to conflict unless the situation is well managed.* (NHS Executive, 1998, para 2.7)

The laudable aim of 'balance' is further echoed in *A national strategy for carers* (DoH, 1999):

> *We want to strike the right balance. By empowering carers we are not taking away any of the rights of the people who need care, nor recognising their needs any the less.* (DoH, 1999, para 13)

In view of these concerns, we therefore examined how the Carers Act is functioning for both carers and the people they are caring for. We looked at the assessment process from both angles, giving each individual an opportunity to be involved and to express their viewpoint.

Research methodology

This report covers the second phase of the *In their own right* project.

The first phase was an overview of 15 local authorities and health authorities in the South West of England, and looked at the effect of the Carers Act on the provision for carers in the different areas. This work is the subject of two previous reports, *View from the top* (Robinson and Williams, 1997) and *A seamless service?* (Williams and Robinson, 1998).

The present report covers work carried out between December 1997 and October 1998, involving fieldwork in five local authority areas in South West England. The five authorities represented a sociogeographical mix, with two urban authorities and two large rural areas. The sample included three new unitary authorities, and two established ones, with a representative proportion (5.8% over all the authorities) of families from minority ethnic groups, mainly in the urban areas.

In each of these five authorities, we carried out two strands of work. The first strand was a records search, to establish the number of carers of people with learning disabilities receiving carer's needs assessments over a period of one year (1 April 1997–31 March 1998), and the kinds of areas covered in these assessments. This work is reported separately (see Appendix B), but a major issue turned out to be the low number of carers who had had a full carer's needs assessment. Of those carers whose relative with a learning disability had had a community care assessment over this period ($n = 157$), only 22% had received a full carer's needs assessment.

Secondly, we aimed to interview carers and 'cared for' people in families who had recently had a carer's needs assessment. Following the interviews with the

carers, the plan was also to interview the care manager, mainly by telephone.

Given the low number of carers who had received a full carer's needs assessment, however, we decided to broaden the focus of our project. We decided to look more widely at the whole process by which carers' needs, and those of the people they are caring for, are assessed in practice. We therefore included carers whose relative had recently had an IPP (service review), and those who were receiving some kind of 'continuous assessment' of carer need.

Finally, we returned after about one year to the families whom we had interviewed, mainly to examine the outcomes of the assessment process.

For further details on the methodology used in this second strand, see Appendix A.

Demographic details

Carers

The final sample for interviews that we analysed, over all five authorities, was 51. Table 1 shows some of the details about this sample. Most of these people were parents of people with learning disabilities, but the sample also included one foster mother, two sisters and a brother-in-law, and one partner. Forty of the people interviewed were women, four were men, and in seven cases we interviewed the parents together.

Table 1: **Details of the carers interviewed**

Age bracket		Ethnicity	
20-29	1	45	White British
30-39	4	1	Asian
40-49	13	2	African/Caribbean
50-59	14	3	White other
60-69	10		
70-79	9		

It is important to note the ages of these carers. Many people were carrying on caring for people with learning disabilities well into retirement.

People with learning disabilities

The people with learning disabilities for whom they were caring were roughly divided into male and female (26 men or boys and 31 women or girls). Their ages were as shown in Table 2.

Table 2: Ages of the people with learning disabilities

Ages	Number of people
Child (16 or under)	11
16-19	8
20-29	13
30-39	18
40-49	7

Note that the total number of people here is greater than the number of carers, since some were caring for more than one person with learning disabilities.

As would be expected, the sample of people with learning disabilities represented a very wide spectrum of ability. We did not apply or ask for any classification, and so it is impossible to give exact figures about levels of ability or independence. The range was from a person with profound and multiple disabilities, self-harm habits and no verbal communication, to someone who travelled and worked independently and who could run a household when left alone over a weekend.

It was very noticeable that parents/carers saw and described their relative as an individual, and primarily as part of the family. The researcher who carried out the interviews frequently met the parent/carer first, and was often surprised when she then met the person with learning disabilities, since the picture given by the carer sometimes appeared to underestimate or overestimate the person's ability. This appeared to be due to the fact that carers talked of the issues and relationships from a family perspective, and had no need to describe their relative in terms of any general classificatory system.

Nine people communicated through non-linguistic means, and had profound physical and/or sensory problems. Thus the meetings with them, as will be explained in Chapter 5, were not structured interviews in any sense. The researcher tried to communicate by following the interests and leads

given by the person him/herself. Observation notes were made, usually immediately after the meeting, relating to the way the person presented him/herself, the kinds of preferences s/he showed, and the impressions s/he gave of satisfaction or non-satisfaction. This methodology was similar to that used by Morris (1998) in her study of disabled children.

The remaining 34 were capable of listening, responding and/or looking, and so more structured interviews could be carried out. We used a large illustrated booklet, with questions, sketches and photographs, and this gave quite a 'safe' structure to the meeting. People were given the choice of whether or not to use the tape recorder, and in fact only six did so on the first round of interviews. The data obtained was analysed according to themes grounded in the data itself. These were discussed with members of a focus group of people with learning disabilities, who advised the project, and were able to point out the important issues.

A representative sample?

The sample of carers in this study was broadly representative of those who had received assessments of carer need and we were pleased that our interviewees included carers from a wide variety of situations, including those:

- whose son or daughter presented behavioural challenges;
- who had recently had a diagnosis for their son/daughter;
- from different cultures, including European and Asian backgrounds;
- who were busy professionals;
- who had more than one son or daughter with learning disabilities;
- who needed support themselves in managing everyday life tasks.

For further details on methodology, see Appendix A.

Structure of the report

From the evidence of our records search, very few carers of people with learning disabilities are receiving formal carer's needs assessments. We can thus conclude that the vast majority of these carers are not in receipt of their rights under the Carers Act.

Widening our focus in response to this discovery, we were able to collect data about the positive and the negative features of the many different situations in which these carers have their needs identified. We were able to go beyond our original focus on carer's needs assessments under the Act, to answer the question: 'What works well for these carers and their families?'

Chapter 2 outlines the themes emerging about carers' situations and circumstances, while **Chapter 3** looks at their own self-perceptions and the roles they take on. Both these chapters are intended to help assessors and others understand carers' situations and desires. Varied though families' circumstances are, many strong common themes emerged that are worthy of consideration in an overall strategy for this group of carers.

Chapter 4 is about carers' views on needs assessments. It includes their opinions on the IPP process, where this is all they had experienced, and it aims to draw out some of the strong and weak points of practice in both these situations. This is in many ways the central chapter of the report, for those who are interested in improving practice.

Chapter 5 is also about the assessment process, but from the point of view of the people with learning disabilities, whom we also interviewed shortly after their own assessments had taken place. We feel it is extremely important to listen to their viewpoint in the debate about carers' needs. This chapter concludes with four case studies highlighting the changes that had occurred for people when we followed them up after one year.

Chapter 6 goes on to look at the important topic of conflict of interests. If carer's needs assessments are lending weight to the carer's perspective, then this may be at the expense of the rights and interests of the individual cared for. This chapter examines disagreements from all three points of view – the carer's, the individual's and the assessor's – and aims to discover how such disagreements are resolved.

Chapter 7 deals with the data we obtained from carers at the follow-up interviews, one year after their assessment. It is about changes in family circumstances, and service provision, over the year.

Chapter 8, also from the perspective of the follow-up visits, deals with the outcomes of the carer's needs assessments, and carers' retrospective satisfaction with the process.

Chapter 9 draws together the threads from many parts of the report, to provide a comparison of carer's needs assessments and IPP reviews, from the point of view of addressing carers' needs. This chapter also looks at record keeping.

Finally, **Chapter 10** gives recommendations to local authorities based on the findings of this report.

2

Carers' situations

Chapter summary

- Of our sample of carers, 37% were caring for another disabled person, as well as the person with learning disabilities.

- A total of 29% described themselves as disabled.

- Despite these facts, most of the carers interviewed had active and involved lives, and were very keen to fulfil other family roles, such as that of grandparent.

- The position of siblings as young carers was seldom recognised, and older people with learning disabilities who were taking on caring tasks for their parents were not supported at all.

- It was found that a career outside the home was very important for the 31% of carers who had a job, and also that community support was very valued.

- It is important that carers' needs assessments consider the whole situation for the carer, including these outside factors.

Being a carer of someone with a learning disability

Our findings about the situations of carers of people with learning disabilities lend weight to a general picture emerging of this group of carers. They are often isolated and under great pressure, feeling that they have to battle for services throughout the life span of their relative with learning disabilities. Similar points are made, for instance, by Beresford (1995), Parker (1994), Twigg and Atkin (1994). Todd and Shearn (1996) emphasise the amount of time taken up by caring, and the effects this has on the stages of carers' own lives.

Grant and Whittell (1999), on the contrary, emphasise the coping strategies that are used by carers, and the aspects of caring that give rewards and hope. Many of these were reflected in the present study. In some respects, carers of people with learning disabilities constitute a unique group, and their situations and perspective are often distinct from those of other carers.

Other responsibilities

Carers of people with learning disabilities are generally 'caring people', and often have additional responsibilities for disabled relatives, elderly parents or even disabled partners. In 19 of the families we visited (37%), the person with the learning disability was not the only 'cared for' person, and in another three the carer had been intensively involved with another disabled family member who had recently died. We met people who were caring for parents with Alzheimer's Disease, who had nursed their husbands or wives during long illnesses, who had more than one disabled child or stepchild, or who had willingly taken on the role of carer for another person with learning disabilities. One carer put it like this:

> *"I've always felt that I have got to do it for someone, it's a duty."*

Not all were driven by such a conscious sense of duty; indeed, many had extra caring responsibilities thrust upon them, simply because they were already available and at home. We met one woman who came from a large family, but whose brothers and sisters had all left her to be the main carer for her elderly mother, because she lived down the road with her daughter who had severe learning disabilities.

What are the practical effects of all this caring? Many interviewees pointed out that the needs of the different people cared for were often incompatible. For instance, someone who has severe physical problems may need nursing care throughout the day and night in case of emergencies. It is then impossible for the carer to go out and about with an active young daughter with learning disabilities, who needs to develop and maintain her social interests.

Many 'caring' situations are not simple. The needs of the person with learning disabilities have to be considered, and also those of the rest of the family, including the extended family. It is also worth pointing out that many of the people we interviewed did not mention their other caring responsibilities until the end of the interview. It is easy to focus entirely on the person with learning disabilities, and carers are used to this focus from many of the professionals they meet. The carers we interviewed did not think that we would necessarily be interested in the fact that their wife had had a heart bypass operation and could not manage stairs, or that their partner had a disabled parent.

Finally, there was a group of carers who had willingly taken on the role of carer, either by adopting a disabled child or adult, or by becoming the paid carer to a second person with learning disabilities. These people were universally positive about their dual role, and often found that the second person was company for their own child. However, it was still vital to them that services were coordinated to meet the needs of the whole family; for instance, short-term breaks had to be arranged for both the 'cared for' people at the same time, otherwise the carer had no real break at all. Similarly, appointments, social work visits and other professional encounters could multiply unless there was some thought put into the family's needs.

Carers' own impairments

Caring is a task that often takes its toll on people's health, and 15 of the 51 carers (29%) whom we interviewed had health problems which they described as disabilities. We did not count old age as a disability; many very elderly carers were remarkably fit and active. However, the presence of disability in this group is very significant if one takes into account the role that these carers are expected to perform, often seven days a week, 24 hours a day, with very few breaks. Many family carers were working with personal health conditions that would warrant sick leave (indeed, long-term sick leave) if they were in paid work.

Impairments included serious back problems, arthritis, and other physical problems, heart problems, acute illness such as cancer, and bone disease. They also included a fair proportion of mental health related problems. Both the physical and the psychiatric problems could sometimes be related to the caring role, and in a few cases the carer felt that these problems were definitely related to the caring work: "It comes partly with the job", [as this carer pointed out].

It ought to be emphasised that if this were the case for a carer in paid work, the person would be pursuing her employers for industrial negligence. Such an option was not open to, or likely to cross the minds of, any of the families interviewed.

As with the carers' other responsibilities, the issue of their own ill-health or impairment was often not mentioned until the latter part of our conversation. One person said to us specifically that she did not have time to think how *she* felt. Yet many carers are aware of the importance of keeping fit, because of the vital role they play with regard to their disabled relative:

"If anything happened to me, that would be it."

There seems to be a real issue here, which assessors need to pick up. Only 29% of the carer or client assessments in our records search across the five authorities had covered the carer's health. Yet it would seem that this is an absolutely vital area, which warrants full discussion and an appropriate service response.

Of the 15 carers who described themselves as disabled, only five had been enabled to start arrangements for their relative's future care. Moreover, in seven of the 15 cases (47% of carers who had an impairment), the carer's own ability to continue caring had not even been discussed in the assessment. This was also true for the five areas, according to record searches, which showed that 71% of carers were not asked about their own health during assessments.

Carers, even those with impairments of their own, did not necessarily wish to stop caring for their relative. Indeed, we met people who were desperate to continue having at least a minimum of caring responsibility, and to maintain the role, particularly in relation to their son or daughter. However, the support needed does have to be carefully worked out when there are multiple impairments in the family.

Carers with active lives

As well as the high proportion of disabled carers, we also met people who had very full and active lives. Indeed, the two groups (disabled and active) were not mutually exclusive.

One woman told of her many outings, involvement in clubs and trips, and the continuing purpose in her life, compared with the lives of many of her neighbours. This was a woman in her late 50s, who explained that:

"It keeps us young."

We met elderly parents who were still very involved in many interests outside the home, and who had active hobbies of their own. Some of these interests were directly related to the business of being the parent of someone with a learning disability (eg organising Gateway Clubs, going on trips and holidays with groups of people, running jumble sales), while others were personal interests (eg cycling, rambling, playing a musical instrument, training guide dogs for the deaf). Indeed, it ought to be said that inclusion of the person with learning disabilities in the local community often happened through the parent's own interests. One woman with profound and multiple impairments attended a local music group with her mother, and was accepted as a part of the group, benefiting from group trips and activities as well as rehearsals.

Meeting this group of carers was a real privilege, and the picture of caring we saw was certainly not all doom and gloom. This was most definitely not a group of down-trodden, disabled, 'only-just-coping' individuals with multiple problems of their own. They were, on the whole, a real bunch of 'survivors' and had a fantastic amount of insight, ability to communicate and real enthusiasm to offer. The very problems encountered along the way often contributed in the end to a positive personality and self-image. One carer, who had become an active lobbyist and campaigner, committee member and professional trainer, said:

"So I have made a choice to take my anger and to be a lobbyist at the highest possible level, as well as locally, and I feel that this way I, with my skills and background, I've been able to get some self-esteem. And it's not just that I've had a bad deal, I think of it as something positive."

Family roles

Assessments need to look at the whole picture for a carer, which includes the role in relation to other family members. In particular, older carers frequently (almost universally) felt it important to fulfil their role as grandparents. Grandchildren were often being looked after, and were sometimes present during our research interviews. Carers acted as babysitters and childminders. As one older carer proudly said,

"My grandson calls me super-gran."

Some parents said that they felt it was particularly important for them to be good grandparents, since this was a way of 'paying back' their other children, who had missed out on opportunities during their childhood, as a direct result of being the brother or sister of a person with learning disabilities.

Even closer to home, the relationship of the 'main carer' with his or her partner was of prime importance. Carers often feel that they do not have enough time to give to this relationship, and several of the people we spoke with said that their partner had different views from them about the caring situation. Others mentioned the fact that they found it impossible to go out together or have common interests, since one of them always had to sit for their disabled relative. It is very easy to forget the perspective of the 'other carer' – often the husband or male partner – who also has needs and deserves recognition for his contribution.

Where the carer had 'taken care' to give time to her main relationship, this was cited as a very positive thing, since the two partners could then genuinely feel that they worked as a team within the family, "... because we are strong. We've got consistency". All too often, carers felt that they had had to develop separate interests, since, as younger parents, they had *never* been able to go out together, which can be an added stress on the marital relationship. However, our interviewees included people who positively valued their relationship, and felt it really important to devote time to it.

The implications for assessment of needs should be obvious: short-term breaks are not just for holidays, they are for the essential ongoing business of partner relationships. For instance, a befriending service, which enables the person with a learning disability to go out for the evening in their own right, without their parents, was a very valued service, since parents were then able to have time just on their own, in their own home.

Young carers: part of the family

If the partner needs to be considered in an assessment, so, of course, do young carers – in this case, brothers and sisters of the person with a learning disability. We found that siblings in these families were *never* being recognised as 'young carers'. Only one child had had a carer's needs assessment (at the insistence of his mother), the outcome of which had been that he was not considered to be carrying out caring tasks.

The lack of recognition of young carers extended to the parents we spoke with. Parents often acknowledged the problems that their other children faced within the family. They recognised that the disabled child was often the focus of attention, and that his/her needs might be incompatible with those of their other children. However, they did not think of their other children as 'young carers'. Given the fact that parents of children with learning disabilities did not use the word 'carer' about themselves, this is hardly surprising.

More importantly, however, most parents did not want to single out any particular child. Many of the parents we met, especially those with younger children, took pains to treat their children equally. They did not want to single out the child with learning disabilities for 'special treatment', but equally they did not want the siblings to feel that they were any different because of having a brother or sister with learning disabilities. Labelling the 'special child' for them was no different from labelling the other children as 'young carers'. It would be tantamount to putting the two types of children in two separate camps, and parents were understandably anxious not to do this.

"It's typical brothers, and he's a typical boy. It's just that he's got a handicap."

"We didn't want to have two kids, and Anna. I have got three kids and a husband. They're all just part of the family."

Efforts to accept individual differences as 'just part of family life' were very common. There was evidence, however, from other carers with older, grown-up children, that support in responding to their needs and reactions would have helped. In one family, one brother had become quite disturbed as an adolescent, and the parents now saw how traumatised he had been as a child, while the other sibling had accepted and met the situation positively, had taken up a career in the caring profession, and was actively helping with her severely disabled brother. People are all different, and this parent reflected that:

> *".. when you are sitting six or seven year olds down, and telling them [about] their baby brother, I don't think as parents you start to comprehend – well, that just goes to prove how differently both of my children took it."*

The wish to be fair to all the children, and not to single out one child, was also possibly linked with their own sense of total responsibility. It is easy for parents to feel that they have to cope entirely with any problems one of their children presents, especially when that child has a learning disability. Their wish not to burden their other children often extended into adulthood, and many parents stressed that they did not want their other sons or daughters to have to care for their brother or sister after their own death.

The perspective of young siblings was generally missing from this study, but there were clearly some adult brothers and sisters who were quite prepared to take on the role of carer. Indeed we interviewed three carers who were in fact sisters of the person with learning disabilities. One of these, who had been brought up with her brother, felt that she had been a carer for over 50 years – a lifetime of caring! Not only had she taken the role of main carer for her brother, with extreme cheerfulness and competence, but she was also caring for her mother with Alzheimer's Disease who lived together with them:

> *"My mother has always been very much against any sort of residential care, even respite care."*

'Keeping it in the family' is perhaps more a thing of the past now, and all these situations were with middle-aged people with learning disabilities. However, some brothers and sisters were providing excellent support for their sibling with learning disabilities, possibly unencumbered by feelings of guilt and responsibility. In one case, the individual

had an extensive family home, split between his various brothers and sister, so that his own independence included the ability to relate to different members of his family, as he chose.

To return to the childhood of these siblings, whether or not the word 'young carer' is appropriate, the needs and views of brothers and sisters must be sought when providing support to families. It is perhaps by opening up channels of communication early on in childhood that later problems can be avoided.

Mutual caring in families

Caring is by no means always one-way. Many people with learning disabilities are caring for elderly parents, or helping out in other ways. Walmsley (1996) has recently drawn attention to this reversal of roles, and it was apparent in at least nine of the families we interviewed too.

One mother told us that she tried to send her son for short breaks into the hostel, since she felt it was good for him to be away for a whole week from home. However, she missed him when he was away, because he does a variety of physical tasks in the home, including lifting and carrying, and gardening:

> *"I mean, Andrew does so much in the house that really he does the dustbins and the garden ... so I miss him."*

Another parent who had a physical impairment herself appreciated her daughter's help with the wheelchair, and a third family described a complex web of interrelated care between three people in the family, including a son with severe learning disabilities.

Other, mainly older, parents, spoke of their son or daughter as providing 'good company', especially when they were left alone and widowed.

> *"I would be completely on my own without Richard, he's such a help. I think I would have gone right downhill, but for Richard. Even from the start, he was there with his company, somebody else in the house."*

Recognition of mutual dependency, however, was very rare. Although parents spoke of the tasks performed around the house, they seldom saw this as implying that their son or daughter was becoming a 'carer' in any sense. They had instead an extremely strong and overriding sense that they themselves were still the carer (in the sense of being 'responsible for') their son or daughter.

In interviews with the people with learning disabilities, we also asked about the help and support they gave to their parents. None of them saw themselves in the role of 'carer', but instead spoke of the tasks they did around the house as if these were part of their programme of learning independence skills. Support and assessment of the needs of this unrecognised group of carers were non-existent, although some day centres are beginning to be aware of the need.

Career prospects of carers

Caring is a career in itself, and increasingly recognised as such both in the literature (Shearn and Todd, 1997), and by carers themselves. One mother spoke to us about her 'right to retire' from caring when she reached retirement age. However, she also expressed the dilemma felt by many carers who have reached this age without ever having had the opportunity to pursue a regular career outside the home:

> *"If I had made a career for myself it would be different. But I have given my life to Sharon."*

She now faced the prospect of Sharon moving on and leaving the family home, and had no sense of what her own role would then be. It was too late, she felt, to start any career interests at her time of life, and she feared the loss of purpose her daughter's move would bring. This insight is, of course, linked closely with the reason for many older carers being quite happy to continue caring for as long as possible, not wishing to 'retire' and putting off arrangements for the future.

However, a career outside the home was of great importance to many people, and 16 of the 51 people interviewed (31%) told us about their careers. It is remarkable when it is recalled that another 15 of the interviewees described themselves as disabled, and a good proportion of all these

people had very active voluntary work commitments. The jobs that carers were doing covered a whole range, from professions such as teaching and social work or senior posts in business, to part-time cleaning or secretarial jobs. We asked more systematic questions about work outside the home in our follow-up interviews.

The difficulties of juggling a job with a caring role are not to be underestimated, and the expected problems were of course mentioned. Some of the people who had retired from paid work had, in fact, done so precisely because of these problems, which included lack of flexibility with hours of work, the inability to meet employers' demands, the necessity to be at home until the 'cared for' person had left in the morning, and so on.

It was also noticeable that people in the lower paid and more menial jobs were more likely to encounter these problems, reflecting a lack of understanding on the part of their employers. In some respects, it was easier to be a mental health social worker, because although these people were in busy and responsible jobs, they at least had understanding colleagues and structures, and a flexible routine.

Why do these carers, then, fight for their right to work and pursue a career? The reasons are fairly obvious. Parents who had full-time caring roles bemoaned the financial situation they were left in when they reached retirement age, receiving the same pension as their peers who had not been carers. No account was taken of the fact that they had been carers for all of their lives, and indeed still were.

> *"I have cared for 33 years for people, no holidays, no breaks, no going home at the end of the day. What is work if it is not caring? And at the end of the day, when I become a retired old aged pensioner, I am not entitled to an old age pension, because they say I have not worked, and paid my stamp. But I have been caring all this time, and that makes you very angry, especially when [I've cared for two people], and you're saving the authorities thousands of pounds. They have very little thought for anything."*

The financial situation is indeed a major reason for working outside the home at every stage, but it is not the only one. Those who had careers were very positive indeed about the support they received from colleagues, often citing their work colleagues as their main source of information, as well as personal support. Work also gives status and fulfilment, which is of paramount importance to many people. One woman, looking back at her earlier life as a full-time carer, said:

> *"Not only did I not have any career, I didn't even have any social status outside of being a carer. And that was so destructive to me."*

The messages that came from these interviews were very clear. Firstly, the right to work must be recognised and backed up with services that make it possible. However, it is not only the services that should respond. Employers generally need to become more aware of carers' needs, and allow flexible hours and working conditions to meet those needs. Our records search over the five areas in this study revealed that only 9% of full or partial carer's needs assessment referred to work issues.

Secondly, the career of caring itself needs to be recognised and given status, as is emphasised in *A national strategy for carers* (DoH, 1999), which suggests that time spent caring will entitle carers to a second pension. Not all carers actually want to pursue an outside career, but they nevertheless should be granted:

- recognition of their skills and contribution;
- breaks and;
- retirement pension.

Support from the wider family and the community

Many of the carers in these interviews spoke warmly of the good relationship between their adult sons and daughters and the son/daughter with a learning disability. Visits to other family members, including grandparents, were very much valued, although in some cases it was quite difficult to maintain these visits without private transport. The isolation felt by the 'main carer' was considerably relieved when he felt that there was a network of family members on whom he could call. For those who did not have this family network, a network of

close friends or colleagues could perform broadly similar functions.

While 'friends or family' were often cited as the main source of support, featuring a long way ahead of official, statutory services, some families were less fortunate. Some had relatives – or more often, branches of the family – who did not understand and support them at all. This was clearly a source of great hurt and breakdown of relationships.

> *"They felt that I shouldn't keep James, and they've never wanted to know."*

The existence of wider family support is a very important factor when considering individual carer needs, and stereotypes can be misleading. One Asian carer in the study, for example, gave us a very revealing picture of the lack of support she experienced, both from her own wider family, and from the Asian community generally. She felt it was easier to go out in an English setting with someone with a severe learning disability than among Asian friends. She said that no one understood her needs in the family, often thinking she was happy when she was barely coping.

Beyond the boundaries of family and friendship circles, there were also mixed responses from the wider community. In particular cases, there were aspects of community that were very helpful, and integration into community activities was very much valued by all families whose disabled family member experienced it. In particular, several carers from different faiths mentioned their church activities and the church community as being invaluable sources of support. Neighbours could also be very supportive: as one parent said:

> *"We know that one another is there for each other."*

Since some people with learning disabilities do become well known in their neighbourhood, carers often had a role to play in getting to know neighbours, explaining the person's needs and methods of communication – in fact, providing informal disability equality training to their neighbours.

However, some families did not enjoy such a supportive neighbourhood atmosphere. There were families who suffered racial abuse from neighbours, and there were many who found it hard to take their son/daughter into the wider ('unknowing') community at all. This was particularly so for those whose relative had behaviour that was unconventional or, indeed, challenging. These parents found that people could become very unaccepting when someone was loud, or exhibited anti-social behaviour. One parent told of the time when she had taken her son out to a fair, and he had become over-enthusiastic about looking into a small baby's pram. The general public, she said, had hardly needed the fair – they were quite ready to stand and stare while she had to cope with his behaviour. Incidents like this can be extremely hurtful, and some parents find that they cannot face taking their son or daughter into situations where they might occur. Indeed, there is a tendency to divide the world into 'special situations':

"... where people are already aware of his position"

and 'outside situations' in the wider community where people might respond in ways that hurt the family. Parents, in particular, desperately want their son or daughter to 'pass' socially when they are out in public places.

Families whose relative has behaviour that does not 'fit in' in any way to community norms especially need support. If it is true that the wider community still needs to learn a lot about supporting and accepting individual differences, then we all need to be part of that change. It should not be left to individual carers and families to fight that particular fight by themselves, because they are precisely the people who will be most hurt by unhelpful responses. Carefully matched befrienders, or support circles, can be a very valuable service in supporting these families, and enabling the individual to access the local community.

* * * * * *

Carers' needs assessments, therefore, need to look very widely, not just at the main carer, but at all the family members, the extended family, the community surrounding the family, and the wider community in which that family lives.

3

Carers' perceptions of themselves

Chapter summary

- The carers we interviewed generally did not describe themselves as 'carers'. This word was reserved for physical caring, and was also associated with paid carers.

- Parents and carers felt that they had had to battle for service provision for their son or daughter, although some did not want to get a bad reputation because of this.

- Self-help and mutual support groups were often not used, for various reasons. Some carers found that the most useful help they got was from other people who had some experience of being a carer. This included carer support officers.

- There was a strong tendency for carers to praise the services, and to align themselves with front-line workers, as they felt that any criticism might lead to withdrawal of vital support.

- Many had difficulty in seeing the person cared for as an adult.

- However, many carers said that the needs of the person they cared for were paramount, rather than their own needs as carers.

Perception of the word 'carer'

Our interviewees tended to identify 'caring' with practical, physical care tasks. Twigg and Atkin (1994), on the other hand, identify more abstract elements, such as 'being responsible for' and Nolan et al (1994) found that it was precisely these more intangible aspects of relationships which were the most important for carers themselves. In practice, the assessment process often finds it easier to focus on measurable, discrete and concrete caring 'tasks'. However, it is more important to understand the carer's subjective interpretation of their situation than to focus solely on tasks performed (Nolan et al, 1996).

To some extent the Carers Act has institutionalised the word 'carer', but it is not necessarily a word that has meaning for those who support people with learning disabilities at home. This is important, since it is hardly likely that people will seek to have a 'carer's needs assessment' if, as Beresford (1995) found, they do not see themselves as carers.

None of the parents of children with learning disabilities thought of themselves as carers. The most typical comment was: "We're just her mum and dad", or even in one case "I'm just a general mum". People said to us sometimes that, even though they were caring, they were "still a mum". This does indicate that people may have a reluctance to accept the word 'carer' since to them it implies that they are no longer a parent.

Many people with whom we spoke associated the word 'carer' with physical caring. For instance, where someone was caring for both a relative with a physical impairment and a relative with learning disabilities, they were more likely to call themselves a carer for the former. One parent spoke about her son like this:

"I think he needs support, but not a lot of looking after."

'Caring' was also associated with taking responsibility for someone. With children, it is accepted as part of the parental role that the parent will be responsible, and so the need to designate oneself as a 'carer' on these grounds does not loom large until a person with learning disabilities reaches adulthood.

One parent of a 19-year-old said that he had only just thought of the word 'carer' at the transition stage, when he realised that:

"He's not going to go off and be independent – he's always going to be our responsibility."

Further confusion is caused by the fact that the word 'carer' is not new to families, since it is also used for professionals who provide paid care (see also Beresford, 1995). One parent said that a carer is "someone you get in when the family can't cope". The mismatch in terminology between professional practice and families' perceptions appears to be a real problem, and could well contribute to the low take-up of carers' needs assessments.

The fighting mentality

If the people we spoke with did not see themselves as 'carers', they certainly saw themselves as 'fighters'. In almost every interview people used images of war or fighting. People had had "battles with social services" over short breaks provision. They had had to "fight the Education Authority" for special schooling, or the right to have people with profound and multiple impairments accepted in day centres. We met carers who had had to fight for their right to Disabled Living Allowance, or had fought for four years to secure an educational psychology assessment that would guarantee a place in residential school. The battles are endless, although many parents (of all ages) did admit that they were tired of fighting.

"The fight is going out of me ... I'm just too tired to fight any more."

Some older parents we spoke with had been part of the parents' movement in the 1950s and 1960s, when there was very little state provision for their children. In order to secure an education, or a right to a day placement, parents had had to join forces in organisations such as MENCAP. They were justly proud at having been instrumental in assuring the right to many services, such as residential support in community housing or day centre provision. They were worried by their perception that younger parents were not joining organisations like MENCAP any more. Parents in general feel that they are advocates for their son or daughter, but parents who are fighters see themselves almost in the role of crusader – battling not only on behalf of their own child, but also for other disabled people – and they were anxious to see the fight continued.

The younger parents we spoke with, however, still felt that they had a lot to fight about, although they were tending to fight these battles alone. Many parents of all ages, who were prepared to challenge the status quo, were aware of the problem of attracting a bad image in the eyes of authorities and service providers, and gaining the reputation of being a 'stroppy parent':

"We were avoided like the plague because we were challenging the system."

Indeed, parents were sometimes not prepared to risk acquiring this reputation, since they thought it might count against them in the allocation of resources.

On the other hand, other more assertive parents felt that their reputation as fighters was the only thing that did help them gain resources:

"The only thing that's made any difference is to get a reputation as someone who's prepared to go to court and win."

The fighting mentality is linked in many cases with the voluntary worker image. For many parents, voluntary activities had become part and parcel of their lives, and had given them a strong sense of purpose over many years. The sense of identity this had given people is not to be underestimated. One mother said it was like: "being in the land of the living again."

Many were still active volunteers, willing or unwilling. Gateway clubs and other evening activities usually rely on volunteers, and we also found volunteers who were helping out with trips and holidays or in day centres. Sometimes parents had to support their own son or daughter in day centre activities, such as swimming, if they were to take part.

Mutual support and self-help

Where parents and carers had banded together for joint campaigning or other activities, there was a lot of mutual support. Sometimes, groups for carers and parents are also set up deliberately to provide this mutual support, and all the parents who took part in any of these groups or organisations felt that they were extremely important and valuable.

> *"When you ring them, you feel they'll understand ... we have all got the same situation. Social workers would not have the time to listen ... it helps you put things in perspective, to know that there are other people with problems."*

However, it must be said that this kind of carer support is not everyone's choice. Some families made a deliberate choice not to get involved, since they felt it would identify them as "a handicapped family". Others were not able to get involved because they lived too far away and could not get to groups, or they found their caring responsibilities took up all the available time.

Some families had also found very valuable support from particular people they came across in services, who happened also to be parents or have experience of being a carer. Carer support officers, for instance, who were often carers themselves, or ex-carers, were able to empathise more fully than other people. They also knew from first-hand experience what parents should do next, what information they needed, and what questions they were *not* asking!

Co-professionals

As we have indicated, we met several parents of disabled children who had taken up professional careers in social work, nursing or teaching. Sometimes this was before, and sometimes after, their caring role started. In either case, they were able to bring a depth of insight and experience to their work role which was invaluable to others.

However, the role of carer is a job in itself, and the skills gained by these people are many and various. One mother, for instance, appeared to have devised better solutions than the consultant for her relative's sleep problems, and the consultant apparently recognised this and treated her with respect. Two other parents were involved in different ways with social services consultation activities.

According to some of the carers we interviewed, they were treated as co-professionals by many of the care managers and service providers with whom they had come into contact. For instance, one mother had a system worked out with day centre staff whereby they both monitored her son's epilepsy. Another parent was the main person to prepare her son for his IPP review meeting, on behalf of the centre. Staff regularly contacted and asked advice from parents, and more than one parent had been involved in providing training to social workers or other professionals.

In contrast, there was another group of carers who were very dissatisfied in this respect. Some health service professionals in particular had failed to take seriously reports of illness or symptoms that later did prove to be real. One young man had suffered serious spinal curvature as a result of his mother not being taken seriously, and another woman had problems with her legs that had not been corrected. As her mother said,

> *"You're given the impression that you don't know what you're talking about ... leave it to the experts."*

Many carers also felt that they were left with all the responsibility of a professional without any of the recognition. This applied particularly to parents of people who presented difficulties to services, through challenging behaviour or by virtue of the fact that they needed extra medical interventions.

Service providers might feel that they are adopting a co-professional attitude by asking the parent how to cope with various problems, but we did see situations where this had misfired, and the parent felt that they were being held to account for their son or daughter's problems. They even felt that their offspring might be excluded from particular provision (eg a hostel for short breaks) if the staff could not manage them. This was very hard for parents to take, when they had to manage unaided for the rest of the time:

"I assumed that the respite was to give us a rest, and if they are saying that Ben is difficult, well I thought it was their job to look after people like this ... Ben is Ben, I can get his drugs changed, but I can't change the way he is."

The role of co-professional, of course, does not mean that parents have all the solutions and expertise, but rather that they would like to have access to professional training and expert advice, in the same way as service providers would have. One of the wishes most commonly expressed in the interviews was for 'expert, professional advice':

"What I would really like is what I would call professional support. Although I know Mark very well, and I can handle most situations, I would like more information about his condition, and what I can do to improve his independence and to improve his communication."

Modesty and the appreciative parent

It is well known (Beresford, 1995) that this group of parents and carers tend to make very modest demands on services:

"All I want is five minutes to myself a day."

"I personally haven't asked for extra help ... it would upset the status quo. All I want is just a couple of days extra respite, otherwise I can cope."

This trend towards modesty seemed to be linked with a tendency to make excuses for service provision. It was precisely the 'modest' carer who was careful to praise the local services that her family did receive, however inadequate they may be.

Time after time, we were told that day centres were doing a very good job really, "considering they were understaffed", and that they were:

" ... all dedicated, wonderful people."

Indeed, more than one carer told us of presents that she gave to staff at Christmas, to show her appreciation of their work. One mother told us that the parents locally were "battling to keep the centre going" and that that was the reason they would not wish to put too much pressure on it. They were often aware of pressures on front-line staff, and they felt a sense of alliance with them, while the people at 'County Hall' constituted the unknown or even hostile force.

However, there was also a strong feeling among some carers that they did not want to tempt fate. The subtext of much of what was said in this vein was that carers have had to fight for what they have got, and were determined not to rock the boat and ask for more. Again, more than one carer explained this attitude quite explicitly:

"I think sometimes there is a general opinion of the majority of carers of disabled people that what they are given is precious ... keep their mouth shut or they might lose it ..."

"A lot of people are of the opinion, we are so glad they take them off our hands, that they are frightened to speak out."

This is far from a rights-based approach, and was not universal. It was, in some ways, the other side of the coin from the fighting spirit that was so evident in some families. However, it can be strongly linked with the sense of responsibility that many parents feel for their son or daughter, and is still very common. People need time and encouragement to work out what would really be a good service. They also need to have the confidence to pursue their rights.

How carers see the person they are caring for

A very common theme in the interviews with carers was their focus on the needs of the person they were caring for. Time and again, people said to us:

> "If the services were right for Jane, I would have no needs myself. As long as she is happy, so am I."

Many carers feel like this, of course, but this particular group of carers – particularly older ones – find it very hard to distinguish their own identities and needs from those of their relative. Indeed, many seemed to assume that their interests and points of view were identical.

This is partly an expression of their dedication and commitment, but it does lead to (or stem from) a view of the individual with learning disabilities as a dependent child. Many parents talked of their adult son or daughter as a child, and there was also a distinct tendency to discount their abilities and skills, as if these did not matter. Some parents were even alarmed when others tended to overestimate the ability of their adult son or daughter:

> "She can't think for herself. I mean, they all think that Jess is quite normal, but she's not really."

Some of the older parents, naturally enough, still used outdated terminology such as 'mentally handicapped'; more importantly, however, there were some who felt it was dishonest to pretend that people had learning disabilities rather than a mental handicap. There was a sense of insider knowledge here; some in this group of parents referred to all people with learning disabilities as 'our people':

> "Our people can never stick at things – they couldn't hold down a proper job."

One of the biggest needs might be for families in general to have more positive images of disability and what disabled people can achieve, and not to feel that they themselves are totally responsible for their children's 'shortcomings'. Such positive images will only emerge when services support individuals adequately to lead adult, more independent lives. The guilt-ridden carer who feels he is 'the only one who can cope' will then be a thing of the past.

Carers' views on their assessments

Chapter summary

- Eight out of 20 carers' needs assessments had been requested by the carer, but five of these were people who were in caring-related professions themselves. Publicity and information campaigns appeared not to have had much effect.

- There was a great deal of confusion about the process of the carer's needs assessment, what it was, and why it was offered.

- The person doing the assessment could be familiar to the family, or new. The most important factors were that they listened carefully, and that they read the records available before the visit.

- The focus of IPPs was on the service user, but carers did sometimes feel included in the process. A focus on the service user's needs was not incompatible with a focus on carers' needs.

- A private meeting with the carer was essential. Good practice included empathy, sensitivity, time and a genuine needs-led approach.

- Carers felt an urgent need for concrete, reliable information.

- Health professionals had very seldom contributed to an assessment of carer's needs, but their perspectives would have been invaluable.

- Planning for the future was a vital and unfulfilled need, especially at the period of transition to adulthood and when the carers were becoming older.

- The importance of a record of a carer's needs assessment was apparent to some carers, but few had had a reliable, clear record.

- Many carers were cynical because of experience of unfulfilled promises.

Methods of assessing carer need

We followed up carers after some kind of assessment had taken place, but this was not always an official *carer's needs assessment*. We also met families where the carer's needs had been taken into account on a continuous basis, and some where the person with a learning disability had recently had a service review (IPP) (see Table 3).

Thus, we are in a position to draw comparisons and lessons from the various types of assessment, both by looking at the same theme across situations, and by comparing one situation (eg an IPP) with another (a carer's needs assessment). In this chapter, we do so from the point of view of the carer.

Table 3: What kind of assessments?

Carers Act	20
IPP	25
Children Act	6

Timing

We found only a handful of carers who had received information from leaflets or other official sources and had then actually requested the carer's needs assessment for themselves. Only one out of the 51 carers we interviewed had found out about carers' needs assessments through the publicity campaign immediately following implementation of the Carers Act, and had pressed her social services department to give her an assessment.

Out of the 20 carers' needs assessments we followed up, only eight had been requested by the carers themselves. Two of these people described how they had to fight for the right to an assessment:

"I had to shout loudly – I basically phoned up the Duty Manager every morning to make sure my request was logged."

Even at the transition stage for their son or daughter (typically, on leaving college) parents had to chase up an assessment themselves. Of the eight carers who had requested assessments, five were professionals in caring, teaching or related careers, and had access to information through their jobs. Only three had requested carers' needs assessments as a result of information they had read, and one of these had heard about the process at an *In their own right* consultation meeting! The other two had gained their information from a CNA leaflet picked up at Boots and a local authority booklet. However, the request based on the local authority booklet did not appear to have resulted in a full carer's needs assessment.

The other 12 assessments had been offered by social workers or other care managers. As we mentioned in Chapter 1, the most common time to be offered an assessment was when a change had occurred in the circumstances, either of the family (eg two families had recently moved into the area) or for the services (eg seven assessments had been offered as a result of a review of provision for short breaks), or

as a result of death or illness of the main carer. Assessments also happened at the transition stage (three cases), when the individual's case was transferred from the Children's Team to the Adult Team. However, even then it was not universally offered.

In children's services, carers' views were sought on an ongoing basis, and there was hardly ever a point at which one could pause and say that a carer's needs assessment had taken place. Parents of children with learning difficulties were neither requesting carers' needs assessments, nor (in any official sense) being offered them.

It is obvious that the publicity campaigns about carers' rights to an assessment of their own needs have not met with great success. Some social work teams had a policy of offering carers' needs assessments at particular moments, but there seemed to be no overall pattern. The general ignorance about the Carers Act among carers echoes the findings from other national surveys (Holzhausen, 1997).

Awareness and understanding of the process

When a carer's needs assessment did take place, how well did the carer understand what was happening? We asked people why they thought the care manager (social worker, or assessor) had come to see them. The picture was one of remarkable confusion, again mirroring the national picture in relation to carers generally.

Unfortunately, the word 'assessment' is all too familiar to many families, whose son or daughter has been subject to assessments throughout their childhood and beyond. In this context, assessments determine whether or not the child has particular educational or developmental problems, and the outcome of assessments in the school years is most often a referral for special educational support.

Therefore it is not surprising that a number of parents felt uneasy about the idea of a 'carer assessment' and entirely misunderstood its purpose. They felt that the assessment would be some process to determine whether or not they were good, competent carers.

It is also not surprising that assessors, in this situation, take care *not* to use the words 'carer assessment' too much: they may try to avoid misunderstandings by saying that they are just coming for a chat. However, the result of this was a general confusion and lack of clarity about purpose.

When asked why the social worker had visited, several carers did not talk about the broad aims of a carer's needs assessment, but thought instead that the visit was to discuss specific problems. These ranged from the disturbed sleep patterns of the individual cared for, to the possibility of finding suitable day placements for their relative. Others felt that the carer's needs assessment itself was separate from the 'user' assessment, but associated the 'carer' part of it simply with filling in the form:

> *"I'm sorry, I fill in so many forms, that I don't remember now whether I did a carer's assessment or not."*

There was also a significant group of carers who had not realised they were having a carer's needs assessment:

> *"The first I knew was when the social worker asked me if I'd like to take part in this research."*

and among these was more than one who still did not know they had had a carer's needs assessment when we visited for the research. Finally, there was a carer who thought she *had* had a carer's needs assessment, and indeed told us all about it, although the social worker later informed us that it had not yet taken place!

Of the carers who were not in relevant professions, only two offered a clear explanation of what a carer's needs assessment was. One person said, for instance, that the worker had come to see them "to catalogue my own needs for now and for the future".

As mentioned above, some carers in relevant professions had prior understanding of what a carer's needs assessment meant, but this was entirely due to their professional role. If a carer's needs assessment is to stand any chance of being successful,

then clearly the assessors must make a priority of explaining to the carer what is happening, why it is happening and what the outcomes might be.

Familiarity with the assessor

In the IPP situation, many carers had known the keyworker who led the review over the years. There was only one case in which a mother had reservations about a keyworker who was well known to her. In all other cases, familiarity was construed as a good thing, for various reasons. Some felt that their own feelings were better understood due to this long familiarity, and all families certainly felt that their relative with learning disabilities had a better chance of being understood by someone who knew them:

> *"Yes, Sandra's very nice, and he has had her for about 18 months I think. She can really talk to our James, and he seems to talk and rely on her a lot."*

In the carers' needs assessments, eight of the professionals doing the assessment were known social workers (or other professionals) who had had contact with the family, sometimes over many years. These carers felt they had not had to repeat things unnecessarily. Five of the six assessments with families of young children were carried out by people who had worked with the family for years. In one particular case, an independent carer assessor was assigned to a carer who knew and trusted her already as a source of support. This was extremely successful.

However, in many cases the assessor was a totally new person. Twelve of the 20 assessments were carried out by people unknown to the carer. Some families liked the fact that this situation gave them a fresh start with someone who was there specifically to concentrate on their own needs. Their attitude, of course, depended a lot on what type of service they received from this new person. Where the assessors were new to the family, it was essential that the new worker:

- should have read the file beforehand, and found out the details of the family situation, rather than asking the carer to repeat the entire history;

- should establish a rapport through good, responsive listening, followed by action.

Given these two conditions, it seemed often to be a positive advantage to have a new worker appear for an assessment. One older mother, for instance, had felt uneasy at first with a new worker who appeared to be so young; however, after a couple of visits, she said:

"I feel really at home with her now ... she's done more for us in the last two months than anybody's done before."

In situations where the outcomes were not so positive, of course, the newness of the assessor was perceived more negatively. Families felt in particular that it had been pointless to fill out record sheets if these had not been read by the assessor. One parent commented:

"Do they put them all through the shredder?"

If records are not read and digested thoroughly before the visit, the carer feels that she is having to start again, and repeat her whole history for each visit, an activity that can soon become frustrating.

Focus of the IPP: carer or service user?

The IPP reviews, held through (and usually at) day centres, are set up to focus on the individual with learning disabilities, and the attention given to carers can be very limited. However, we followed up these situations, because for many families it is their one regular source of contact and support. We ought to mention here that the IPPs we followed up were only those in which a carer had been involved, and there may well have been others where carers were not involved.

It also ought to be emphasised that many centres would not easily be able to provide many of the positive features of IPPs discussed below, as they require funding and often additional staffing. Many of the features appreciated by carers were made possible only by the goodwill of individual members of staff.

Many of the carers interviewed found it helpful and understandable that the IPP process focused on their relative: this was a familiar and unthreatening situation, whereas they had difficulty in identifying their own needs. "I have no needs" was a common theme.

When carers talked about being involved and listened to, in the context of an IPP, they often meant that the day centre staff shared their views on what the individual with learning disabilities ought or ought not to be doing. For instance, one carer had made sure the day centre staff did not allow her daughter to try and establish a relationship, another had requested that her diet be regulated in a certain way, some had asked for epileptic fits to be monitored and recorded.

Even more frequently, the picture was one in which the day centre staff used the IPP opportunity to talk to the carer about what *she* was required to do at home, in order to carry on the aims and goals established in the centre. This could include encouraging the individual to do household tasks, using Makaton signs for communication, or encouraging punctuality.

In other words, the relationship between day centre staff and carer could be seen as a 'co-professional' one, with the power swinging sometimes towards carer, sometimes towards staff.

Where, then, was the focus on carer's needs in all this? And where, indeed, was the service user's voice? There were examples of good practice in our interviews, where both carer and service user were given a voice. Where a review was really user-focused, then it could also serve the carer very well.

The best practice in focusing on the user's needs was seen where there was thorough preparation with the service user. In two cases, this had clearly happened, even though in both these instances the user had considerable communication problems. In both cases, the centre had thought carefully about accessibility issues, and had made very good use of photos in preparing the person to think about his activities and what he preferred. In one case also, there had been good use made of Makaton symbols in relation to the photos. Both these people, despite their communication problems, were able at our research interview with them, to tell us in a meaningful way about their IPP meeting.

Not everyone will need the same approach, but it is important that time is given to individual preparation, so that the service user's presence at the meeting is not just an embarrassment. More than one carer said that they felt uneasy about talking about their son or daughter in front of him, and felt s/he should not be there. By contrast, one carer whose son had had an assessment for Independent Living Fund money, gave the following account of a really user-focused process:

"In an ideal world, that's how any assessment should be, and it should be asking the person what they think they need, and then giving them the power to do what they think they need, and what they want."

The best practice in focusing on *carer's* needs in the IPP was seen when day centre staff had taken the trouble to prepare the carer before the actual meeting. In one case, parents had brought up their worries about their son taking up paid employment, because they felt they might then lose all their own financial security and benefits. Since the keyworker was aware of the parents' worries, she arranged for a benefits adviser to be at the meeting, and this meant that the parents' issues could be properly discussed.

In other cases, keyworkers had managed to visit the carer at home, although they did not have the staffing to provide this sort of service as a matter of course. In more than one case, the IPP was actually held at home: this could help to ensure a carer focus.

More often, however, the carer felt involved simply because the day centre staff were very familiar with the family, and were in regular contact throughout the year. This meant that carers felt their situation and needs were understood, and that the IPP was simply a formal way of recording this and bringing it all together. In three cases, the IPP had been the vehicle for discussing residential provision with families. In all these cases the issues concerning the person with learning disabilities moving out of the family home had been successfully discussed.

Thus we had mixed evidence of the carers' experiences of the IPP. Comments fell roughly into three camps:

Centred entirely on the individual with learning disabilities (15/24)

"It was all to talk about Robbie's needs. Ours were sort of non-existent."

"It was centred on Rosie, not me. I am very much the bystander."

"We sit back in a corner and shut up."

Centred on the needs of both the individual and the carer (5/24)

Some carers spoke about their needs being intertwined with those of their son or daughter:

"It's part and parcel of the same thing."

Centred on the carer (4/24)

A few carers found that the IPP review was a good opportunity to have a chat with trusted people, and to bring up real needs at home (eg for short-term or emergency breaks) with people who really understood and knew the individual.

It also ought to be noted that, without adequate preparation, this third model can become a form of collaboration between carer and day centre staff, in which they talk *about* the individual, and make decisions on his or her behalf, without really separating out the issues of carer need and individual need. Examples would be where the carer sees the IPP as a time to tell the centre that his son should not be allowed to walk home on his own, or that his daughter should not be given ideas about jobs outside the day centre.

Focus of the carer's needs assessment

The carer's needs assessment, as part of a full care management assessment or review, should recognise that the carer has independent needs, and that these should be looked at separately from the needs and wishes of the individual, so that the resulting care plan can take account of both. It should go without saying that carers' needs assessments, at least, are carer-focused. However, this was not always the experience of the carers:

> *"He came to see me about Mary's needs, it was not about me at all. No one has ever spoken to me about my needs."*

We asked carers how the assessment had taken place, and in nearly all instances, the social worker (or other worker) had seen the main carer individually, often on more than one occasion. Unfortunately for some, it had proved impossible to find a time and place with the carer when the 'cared for' individual was not there.

From the carer's point of view, it also mattered whether or not their partner was involved. Many of the 'main' carers had a spouse or partner, and felt they needed time to discuss things from their point of view without their partner there. This did not mean they did not want the assessor to see the partner too, but they wished the discussions to be separate. In other cases, assessors had also visited other (adult) sons or daughters separately, or even grandparents. All of this, of course, takes time, but given the often complex situations, involving many years of caring, one visit is unlikely to provide an adequate understanding or lead to an appropriate service response.

We found no cases where the carer had used an independent advocate of her own during the assessment process. However, the assessor can in some respects become a kind of advocate, as had happened for the most 'satisfied' carers.

Carers appreciated a genuine needs-led approach, rather than being presented with 'a tick-list of services'. In one case, the assessment had been carried out by a separate assessor (a carer support officer). In two other cases, the social worker had managed to disentangle herself from the issues surrounding ongoing service provision and to focus entirely on the carer's needs.

However, information and access to services were also issues, and the role of a carer support officer who is not the 'care manager' is a sensitive one. It is

important that their role is acknowledged and respected, so that their recommendations carry authority.

This group of carers were not forthcoming about their own needs. They were not used to thinking in those terms, and as parents, they often still felt totally bound up in their son's or daughter's lives even after they reached adulthood. Therefore a good carer's needs assessment must enable them to 'open up'. Carers varied in the extent to which they felt they had been listened to and respected, the two most extreme comments being:

> *"I felt a sense of her relief as she walked out of the door – thank god she does not have to live this life."*

> *"She encouraged me to say what I wanted too. She encouraged me to not feel bad about having needs and wants and desires.... That was the other nice thing about it, just being able to talk about me, and whinge and moan, and feel sorry for myself and all the other things that you do."*

This second case was one in which the assessor had caring experience herself, and was not the care manager for the disabled relative.

To summarise, then, however the assessment takes place, these are the lessons learnt from listening to carers.

* A carer focus is not incompatible with a user focus. When the carer feels confident that her relative has got a voice, and is really listened to, then she can relax and speak about her own needs.

* In order to provide the best conditions for this 'carer focus' to happen, the assessor needs to see the carer personally, and probably needs to take time to see her more than once, or visit other members of the family too.

* The approach which carers seemed to appreciate most was one of advocacy, where the assessor is really disentangling himself from service issues, and enabling the carer to talk freely about needs.

* The model of providing a separate carer assessor, perhaps through a carer support centre, appeared to work very well, and perhaps more authorities could benefit from this practice. However, if carer support officers are given the task of

providing carers' needs assessments, it is important that they have an authoritative role which is well understood by the social work teams.

Scope of the assessment

Service reviews, such as IPPs, are generally more limited than full care management reviews. They are set up to look at the individual's programme within the centre, and so any issues which involve other (or potential) services can be difficult to handle adequately.

Many carers realised this, and most reported that the IPP was "just about the centre and what happens there". They often felt that it was "self-perpetuating", since each review meeting was closely tied to the previous year's goals, and it was built on a developmental or skills model, so that for the carer it appeared to follow on directly in the educational mould.

It was possible, on occasions, for the scope to widen a little, and some centre managers were deliberately trying to provide this more comprehensive service to families. As indicated above, one of the keys to broadening the scope of the IPP is to be able to give adequate preparation time in talking with the carer as well as the service user. Not all centres, of course, would be able to do this with their current roles and funding.

However, the following were other features that were appreciated by families.

Information and contact with other services available

Day centres were often invaluable as a central contact point for general service information. However, most centres which hold such information seem to do so purely by chance or because of the personal experience of individual managers. Carers often felt that they themselves knew more about services than the centre did. Perhaps, then, centres should tap into this source of expertise in their inhouse training.

The presence of other professionals from outside the centre at the meeting

Invitations to IPPs, of course, are at the discretion of the service user, but we met no one who was averse to inviting useful people to their IPP, whether they already knew them or not. Such people could include college staff, social workers (one carer commented that hers "always comes with her chart"!), benefits advisors, staff from the local hostel for short-term breaks and different therapists. The value of a meeting with all these people present is debatable and most service users would not like it. However, additional professionals who had been present had always provided useful new perspectives for the whole family.

Exactly the same issues were discussed in relation to carers' needs assessments, and as a general rule, the wider the scope of an assessment, the more it was appreciated. For some carers, for example, the main issue was housing, yet the social worker often said that this was not their concern. No individual professional can know everything about everything, but there must be a commitment to providing an easy and direct channel of information to carers. The frustration felt by families was well expressed in the following comment:

> *"It would be good to have a whole definitive list of information. It all seems to come in dribs and drabs, and none of it seems to connect up. You don't know what's private and what's state, and what's not worth worrying about because it's got a 10-year waiting list."*

Even carers who were in related professions did not necessarily know about local services. For instance, a former coach escort did not know about an accessible transport service, even though she had lived in the area for 39 years. Equally, a mother who was a community nurse said that the social services team always imagined that she would know when to shout if she needed anything. She said, "this is not always as easy as it sounds!"

An assessor taking on a carer's needs assessment must be seen as a real channel for other services. For instance, it is less than useful, as one carer said, when the Children's Team does not know about Adult Services, or vice versa. Health and social services need to know in some detail about each other's services, and information about education policy and provision is also vital at all stages. Breakdowns in communication mean breakdowns in knowledge for the carer, and all too often the carer herself is left to find out and chase up information.

"... the impetus for finding things out always comes from me. I have to 'phone them, and say: what's happening?... It is still very frustrating not to know, and to help Richard plan for what is going to happen to him."

Good practice was when the carer was not only given direct and comprehensive information, but was given it in a concrete way. This could mean that the social worker had taken the carer and the individual to see various facilities, or had made direct contact to fix appointments for the carer and the individual. It meant not just leaving a list of names and phone numbers, but fixing appointment times to discuss outcomes, so that a definite framework for the process was established. As this satisfied customer said:

"Because I didn't know a thing about X, I didn't know there was such a place existed. Apparently there's several [work places for her son] that she told me about."

Health

Of the 51 carers we interviewed, only one had had a health professional actually involved in their own needs assessment. In this case a physiotherapist had been called in to do a detailed assessment of need, for both the individual with learning disabilities and the carer, who had a physical impairment herself. This was extremely valuable, as it indicated the range of support she would need in order to care for the individual at home. It was fed directly into the carer's needs assessment and led to some appropriate services being provided.

Health professionals, such as speech therapists or physiotherapists, were sometimes invited to IPP meetings, if they were involved or likely to be involved with the individual client, but health involvement in assessing carers' needs was generally non-existent. The two sets of professionals did not appear to interrelate unless they were part of the

same Community Learning Disability Team. In such contexts, these professionals were not there for the carers, but were very much focused on the people with learning disabilities, so that aspects of the carer's health were easily overlooked.

Plans for the future: transition and beyond

The major and most pressing concern for all the carers we interviewed was the topic of future care for their relative. When asked whether they intended to continue caring for their son or daughter, nearly everyone expressed extreme worry and uncertainty, and this clearly dominated much of their thinking:

"Us parents think about that all of the time ... when we are no longer there."

The topic of 'the future' loomed especially large, however, at two stages in the caring career. The first was during the process commonly called 'transition', when the child is becoming an adult, and the family is moving from child services to adult services. The second stage was when carers were starting to realise that they could no longer continue caring, perhaps due to ill-health, or old age, or possibly also because their son or daughter wished to move on.

Reports of carers' needs assessments at the transition stage were not very positive, due to a number of factors.

Parents who had become used to relying on statutory school provision suddenly found themselves faced with a whole new world of adult services to sort out, for which they were often ill-prepared:

"... you spend their whole childhood going from one year to the next, in the secure knowledge that there is the school to go to, but the moment you get to the end of school, and the end of college, there is like this chasm that is yawning there, and you haven't a clue what is going to happen. It's really quite frightening."

The 'handover' from child to adult services was seldom experienced as a seamless transition, and more than one parent reported that the respective social workers appeared to know little about each other's fields. Several parents also found that it was they themselves who had to chase up the relevant professionals, in order to put the 'transition' process in motion. This was particularly so when the young person had a full-time college placement. Although college courses were nearly always appreciated, parents did not always know exactly when the course would finish. Funding for the college place tended to go from year to year, so it was hard for parents to plan ahead.

At a more fundamental level, the whole idea of 'becoming an adult' seemed nonsense to many parents. Adulthood seemed irrelevant to parents, since it did not mean that their son or daughter could manage their own affairs:

"He still needs help and assistance."

The idea of adulthood also brought with it issues of vulnerability and the realisation for many that their son or daughter was not ever going to reach the same level of independence as their other children:

"I mean when they are at school you know where they are, what they are doing and all that, and you can encourage that. But now she is adult, there's going to be work, there's going to be accommodation, the problems, the real problems have only just started. School kids are easy to cope with, but now what?"

Given these worries and their extreme insecurity, parents did not take kindly to an assessor who suddenly came to visit and insisted on treating their 18-year-old as an autonomous adult! The whole idea of adulthood and what it entails needs very careful preparation for all parties, so that misunderstandings do not occur. In particular, the carer's viewpoint is vital in planning at this stage, and schools and colleges need to be an integral part of the planning process.

One carer told us that her son, who was away at residential college, had been asked about his future plans. He said that he wished to go and live at home with his parents, and so this was put on his school review. When the mother telephoned to say "Why haven't I even been asked?" she was told "Well, it is his wish". Other carers said that the college courses had given their son or daughter

unrealistic expectations of what might be available after college, in particular by talking about open employment. They felt that this type of dishonesty had led to grave disappointments when the young person had been given no real help in gaining employment at the end, and had ended up at the day centre.

At this stage parents and young people need precise information about what is available in terms of residential accommodation, day activities and employment. Furthermore, it is not enough just to leave parents with telephone numbers to follow up. The idea of a day centre, for instance, might be quite terrifying to a family who is used to school and college provision. Indeed, parents told us of being suddenly faced with an institutional atmosphere and a crowd of people with disabilities, many of whom appeared far more disabled than their own son or daughter. At this stage, more than any other, both the young person and their parents need role models. Mentoring schemes, where an older disabled person is put in touch with a young person with learning disabilities, can be very helpful in this respect, and family-to-family schemes could also be valuable.

Information is one of the keys to a good carer's needs assessment at every stage, and this study lends weight to the view that future plans need to be talked about openly all along.

Many parents do indeed intend to carry on caring for their son or daughter as long as they can. A common theme was that of "putting the future on hold", exemplified by the following comment:

"You can't make arrangements, can you, really? I will carry on for as long as I can."

Many parents felt that all they could do was carry on for as long as possible, and leave the rest to chance (or the authorities). There was sometimes a blind faith that someone official would step in and do *something* when it was needed. A feeling of duty was also linked with the idea that the parent was the only one who could cope:

"She's my daughter, and I will care for her if necessary throughout the rest of her natural life."

The 'carrying on coping' mentality, however, was increased by a generally profound ignorance of supported living options, and the life-style available to people who moved out of the parental home. Some families had had a single negative experience of residential provision, at some point in the past, and this led them to say:

"There is no other option, because what is there for people?"

The greatest need is for information and definite future planning, even when families still wish to continue caring. This might include visits to different types of facility with a social worker, so that both the family and the person with learning disabilities can make an informed choice about what is likely to be available. All too often it seemed that the carer had been asked about her intentions, had responded that she intended to carry on caring, and had not been seen again until there was some kind of crisis.

Records of assessment

It was interesting that the families we visited could nearly always find and show us the record of their last IPP assessment, which they often had filed away with all the others over the years! However, they were seldom so confident about the record of their carer's needs assessment, or even their care plan. Since some carers had filled in the carer's needs assessment form themselves, often without the presence of the social worker, they did not attach much importance to this record as a legal or binding document.

The force of a written record, however, was apparent to some of the carers. They were aware that if something was written down (eg that their daughter needed one:one support) then it was more likely that they would get it. In a couple of cases, carers were very aware that the carer's needs assessment could be a useful document for them in obtaining their rights, and they had taken trouble to ensure that it was accurate. One carer had experienced a reluctance on the part of the social services department to actually produce a written record of her carer's needs assessment:

"The social worker came and did it with me, and they said that [the form] couldn't be completed until they had whatever, and they are still requesting the same information over and over again ... they are still looking for excuses not to provide the service – I know what they are doing."

The way in which assessments are recorded is very important, and is returned to in Chapter 9.

Promises, promises

However good the assessment, or the carer's satisfaction with the process, the whole endeavour is only really valuable if it does lead to action. Nearly every family with whom we spoke had previous experience of promises that had been made and not kept. This can lead them, of course, to be very sensitive to this aspect of practice, and also very cynical:

"It's all very well saying something, but saying it and then forgetting it is worse than not saying something at all."

Among the unkept promises spoken of were:

- holidays
- supported employment
- adapted shoes
- Mobility Allowance
- family link short breaks service.

As one carer pointed out, people would understand if the worker came back and explained why the particular service was not available, or why she had not been able to sort things out. Often, however, the promise seemed to be linked to a particular individual, who then changed jobs. In most cases of broken promises, the person who had promised the service had never been heard of since:

"You think you have got a good social worker and then he leaves and he is doing something higher up, and he still hasn't done anything he said he would."

Service provision also suffered from the same process of attrition, and carers spoke of services such as a well-woman clinic that 'fizzled out', physios that 'wandered off' and befrienders who disappeared. The resulting cynicism about the carer's needs assessment process was well phrased by the following mother:

> *"I can honestly say that having had a carer's assessment has not made a blind bit of difference in my case."*

The final phase of the study enabled us to go back to the carers we interviewed after one year, in order to see how far the promises that were made to them were kept. Their views on the usefulness of a carer's needs assessment were coloured by these outcomes (see Chapter 8).

5

Views of people with learning disabilities

Chapter summary

- Very few people had any real understanding of what a needs assessment could mean for them, in terms of future planning and choices about their own lives.

- Where people had one:one meetings to discuss their needs, these really helped them to express themselves, and to be heard.

- Most people understood very well that their carers had needs too, and they respected their carers' rights to have an assessment of their own.

- There was a need for advocacy. Sometimes a new, fresh person can be a better and more objective advocate, although time is needed to get to know the person.

- Accessibility of written records could be greatly improved.

- Four people with learning disabilities, who were re-interviewed, told us about changes in their lives since their assessment a year previously:

  › greater independence had led to better relationships with their carers;

  › they had made new friends, which was important for them;

  › each of these four people had made different occupational choices, but none had moved into ordinary paid jobs;

  › new opportunities for independence had given increased self-respect.

- Regular reviews of any new arrangements are needed.

Interview methodology

Our aim was to meet with all the young people and adults with learning disabilities over the age of 11 in the 51 families who took part in the project. This amounted to 45 individuals in all. They formed a very disparate group, and ranged from people with no verbal skills to those who could reason and argue about the assessment process. Therefore, what counted as an interview varied according to the person being interviewed.

Only 34 people could take part in anything resembling a formal interview. However, when we were not able to conduct a formal interview, we made notes of our own about what we had done together, and how the person appeared to be.

It was always valuable to meet people however difficult it was to communicate with them. For instance, in one meeting with a person with no verbal communication skills, we had a short interlude of listening to music together, and he showed the researcher how he could guide her hand with his toe, to turn a tape recorder on and off. In another case, the young person greeted the researcher by allowing her into her space, to help her drink from her cup. All these experiences were valuable, since they gave clues about the needs and skills of the person, and their unique personality and preferences.

Of the 34 people who did respond to interview questions, six participated in tape-recorded interviews, although some of the other interviews also contained some in-depth answers and observations. In some cases, brief answers (yes/no) were combined with non-verbal information to give a fuller picture of preferences. For instance, one man insisted on the interview being conducted in the corridor of the day centre, and for each question he came up to the researcher, listened to what was asked, looked at the drawings (see next paragraph) and whispered his answer before walking off again.

The interview schedule was written in large print, with picture sketches and photographs (where available) of the assessor, and the key service places in the individual's life. On the whole, this was a successful procedure, although the danger was that some people saw it as a test that they wanted to pass, asking afterwards if they had done well. However, taken as a whole, the interviews do give an interesting and consistent picture, and there were certainly some individuals who had great insight, speaking not only for themselves but also for others in their position.

Understanding of the purpose of assessments

Of the 45 people we met, only seven people with learning disabilities in this study expressed some basic understanding of what their assessment was about. Some, of course, were not capable of expressing their ideas about the purpose of the assessment. Even so, the number of those who did understand at some level was extremely low.

It will be recalled that there were at least two types of assessment in the study, namely IPPs (service reviews) and full community care assessments. There were also instances where the individual had

been seen regularly, but had not had a formal assessment of any sort. Six of those who did understand were talking about IPP (review) meetings, and one had not really had a particular assessment, but had a good understanding of the social worker's role in her case.

Typical comments that were taken to represent understanding of the IPP were:

> *"It's to do with my work ... to see what's happening ... they're about my programme."*

This means that not a single person who had had a community care assessment understood what it meant and what the implications were for themselves. Since the sample included some quite able and verbal people, particularly at transition stage, this is quite worrying.

Many people, in both the IPP group and the community care assessment group, had focused on particular issues of the assessment, and saw these as the sole reason for the process. These issues were quite varied:

> *"It's to go to another house [ie for me to find a place to live] ... it's part of his job to find a place."*

> *"She came here to talk to me about the farm work."*

> *"I told him about my problems ... about being bullied at college."*

Even more worrying, many people in the IPP system saw their IPP as a method of controlling and monitoring their own behaviour, and talked about the IPP as seeing "how I'm behaving, and not upsetting people", or "to see why I got on better, how I'm doing". They tended to see other people in the role of judges and controllers of their behaviour, and they felt that they had to live up to certain standards. It was clear from the keyworker and carer interviews, that this was indeed the way that many IPPs were set up, with progress reports from all the staff members working with each individual. In this situation, it would be hard for the individual to feel that they had a voice, and could discuss their preferences for future options, either within a day centre or outside.

There was only one person in the whole sample (51) who had an idea that the assessment process was a time when he could express ideas about future needs and concerns. Even for him, the IPP was primarily a way for people to see "what you've been doing at work", but he did add:

"And plans for the future as well."

Being listened to

Despite the general lack of awareness of what an assessment could mean for them, 22 of the 34 people who responded to interview questions did affirm that they were happy that they had been listened to. Among these 22, of course, there were undoubtedly a number who said 'yes' because they felt that was what would please the interviewer. The more revealing answers were among those who were not sure about being listened to. They often said things like:

"I thought so – it's hard to tell."

Three people pointed out that the worker had mainly talked to their carer, one of these saying that the worker is "sometimes on my mum's side", and another person telling us in detail where the worker had sat in the room:

"He didn't sit down with me like you're doing ... he sat at the table with my mum."

One man said:

"I try to say something, and then I forget what I'm going to say."

This points to the difficulty many people have in speaking up for themselves, particularly at a meeting such as an IPP review. It is hard for anyone, but must be even harder for those who are not used to being listened to, or having to think for themselves, and who may also lack skills and self-confidence. It is especially important, for this reason, that the individual has a chance to talk privately with the person doing the assessment, whether this is an IPP or a full assessment.

Only 12 people could remember having a private meeting with the keyworker or social worker. (This may well be a slight under-estimate, due to problems of recall.) In 10 of these 12 cases they felt happy that they had been listened to, and so it was obviously time well spent. Six had talked privately to their day centre keyworkers before the IPP meeting. In two of these cases, the private preparation for the IPP had been particularly successful, with one keyworker enabling the individual to prepare a picture booklet of photos relating to his preferred activities, and the other keyworker working out with her client what she wanted her to say about the client's wish to take paid employment. This client said that:

"She was helping me speak up."

In full care management assessments, it was interesting that the assessor did *not* always see the individual on a one:one basis. Where the assessor saw the family as a whole, or the parent/carer was present, the individual understandably had the impression that s/he was *not* the focus of attention, rather that the carer was speaking for him/her, or indeed that the whole process was centred on the carer.

It is also interesting to note that there were a number of issues and views brought up by individuals during the research interviews, which had obviously not been mentioned, or taken seriously, during the assessment. These issues usually came up towards the end of the session, when both parties had got to know each other a little. For instance, one person talked about her fear of dying, and her wish to have a rest from working every day. Another man said "the problem is this place [the day centre]" since other clients hit him, although he said at the end:

"I will carry on going to High Ridge in my life. It's my life."

A third individual hinted at past abuse at home, and a fourth person talked of her unhappiness that none of the young people in her area seemed to like her. None of these issues had been recorded in the record of assessment, nor indeed were they mentioned by either the carer or the assessor in their interviews with us. They might well be considered to be too sensitive for airing at the IPP meeting itself, but this really only underlines the case for a private one:one time, to really focus on the individual, so that views and needs can be fully taken into account. There is also a need for training to enable assessors to find ways of bringing such issues into a wider arena.

Feelings about the carer's needs and mutual caring

After talking about their own assessment, we asked individuals whether they were aware that the assessor had also talked with their carer about his/her own needs, and what they felt about that. This was probably quite a difficult question to answer, since many people with learning disabilities are possibly unaware that their carers have needs of their own. There were indeed a number of non-committal answers, such as:

"Alright ... that's OK, I don't mind ... I think that's OK."

A few answers also indicated that the individuals had not understood the question at all.

However, there was a surprising number of people who really did have an understanding of their carer or parent as a separate person, with needs and problems of their own. Fourteen people gave answers that indicated a real sympathy with their carer's needs, and they were universally in favour of their carer having a separate time and attention for their own assessment. These are some examples of their comments:

"She needs a break. That's why I go into the hostel from time to time ... she [the keyworker] can see what my mum wants ... it's a good idea for her to sort things out with my mum."

One young man said that he "worries about his mum", and another young woman often acted as a listening ear herself, but was not there all the time to help her parent. This is why:

"I think that it's important for my mum to have someone to talk to and tell her problems."

Far from objecting to their carers having their own assessments of need, the overwhelming impression was of a group of people who were really considerate and caring about their carers! As noted above, at least nine of the families were in situations where the person with learning disabilities was helping their carer at home. Some helped their carer with basic physical tasks (eg getting in and out of the bath), and others were there to help if their elderly parent was taken ill. More commonly, they reported helping in the garden and with lifting and carrying. However, none saw themselves in any sense as taking on a caring role. Caring was associated with taking responsibility, and this was perceived as the parent/carer's role. In the words of one individual, when talking about her 'carer':

"I think there should be more input, to help X. He lacks a lot of things, and he deserves more. Carers do need a lot of support ... if things go wrong, it all seems to come back on him."

Familiarity of assessor

In all the cases of IPP reviews, the keyworker who led the meeting was a known and trusted person. Very occasionally, there was a keyworker who was not popular with the particular individual, and there were cases where the keyworker had been changed at the request of the person. This was never the case with care managers, who were much less familiar figures for their clients.

Social workers and others who came to do assessments at home were often 'new' and unfamiliar faces, and this was broadly seen as unhelpful by the individuals themselves:

"It was the first time I saw her. When you've got a new social worker, it's like 'who is she?' I'd like to get to know her better. When you've got a new social worker, it's hard to tell her everything. The old one knew everything; the new one says she does, but she doesn't."

It does take time to get to know a person, so that they feel free to express their real concerns. This is particularly so with people who find verbal communication hard, and, for reasons beyond their control, care managers often find it very hard to find time to get to know their clients well.

As with the carers, however, one could argue that a fresh look at a person could be helpful. Keyworkers who have known both client and carer for many years may think that they already know all there is to know about what a person thinks, and what their preferences are. As the examples above show, there is clearly a need for advocacy, so that the individual is really listened to and taken seriously. The day centre staff may be far too used to managing the person's behaviour, and helping him or her to conform and integrate. The care manager may come in to see the family, and not really have time to get to know the individual. Despite the plethora of staff and services surrounding these people, they often lack anyone who will really listen to their own viewpoint in an unbiased way, and encourage and support them to speak up.

Understanding

If the assessment is to be about the individual's needs and preferences at any level, they need to understand it. Accessibility means different things for different people, and indeed there was one person who said she felt rather insulted when people asked her whether she could understand things or not. However, for the vast majority of the people with whom we spoke, accessibility and comprehension were important issues.

Accessibility includes verbal and other forms of communication. Two of the people we interviewed relied on signing in combination with other means of communication – one person was a Makaton user with a preference for making up his own signs, and the other understood many Makaton signs, and also used an electronic communication board. Day centre staff, on the whole, knew their clients well and were able to take account of their verbal communication needs, but it is obviously also important that care managers who visit these people learn how to communicate with them. One profoundly disabled young man had a form of language of his own, which included physical touching and interaction through music and sounds. It was not at all evident that any communication at this level had taken place between him and anyone

who was assessing his needs. If it had occurred, it was certainly not seen as important enough to record anywhere.

In this study, we cannot report on the communication that took place during assessments, since we were not there to observe it. However, what is left after an assessment should be the record, and we were interested to see whether or not this was available and understandable to the individual.

One person graphically described their record of assessment thus:

> *"It's just a pile of paper with lots of squares – tick this, tick that."*

This is how much of the paperwork must appear to the people who are the focus of it. Even a quick glance at most of the records of which we were able to obtain copies confirmed that the language used was not easy to understand. For instance, one individual who showed me the record of his IPP said he could read, but was rather stumped by the phrase:

> *Needs to participate more, verbally.*

There are well documented ways now of writing plain English, or of illustrating with symbols or pictures according to the ability and preference of the individual. Unfortunately, as a direct result of not having access to the printed record of assessment, many people depend on their carer to read it to them. This makes it very hard for any kind of confidentiality to be maintained, and would militate against any private concerns of the individual being recorded.

One IPP record that we obtained for the study was clearly successful, and could act as a model. It was printed on a sheet with an established set of symbols that had been worked out by the social services department. This meant that the format was familiar to the individual. In addition, however, his own strengths and needs, activities and goals were illustrated by means of photos that he had chosen and talked through with his keyworker. The end result of this was that, despite having very little verbal expressive ability, he was able to tell us meaningfully about what happened at his IPP meeting, and what he felt about it.

Follow-up interviews with four people with learning disabilities

We did not seek to re-interview all the people we had met during the first phase of the research, but only a small number for whom there had been significant changes (*n* = 6). Four of these people could tell us about the changes that had occurred for them, and it is these examples that are discussed here. They illustrate what can happen for people as a result of an IPP, or a full community care and carer assessment.

Table 4: **Assessments and outcomes for individuals with learning disabilities interviewed in the follow-up phase**

	Type of assessment	Main service outcome
Jane	IPP	Referral to social worker
Marilyn	Community care	Move to new residential home
Fred	Community care	Started two days a week at a workshop for woodwork training
Julia	Community care	Started full time at an employment training centre

Note: All names have been changed.

All four of these people told us that they thought their assessment had helped things for them. Jane had not had any significant provision of services, as the other three had done, but she said that her IPP was useful, as it "helped me to think about the future". Both Fred and Julia said thoughtfully that their assessment did help, but Marilyn only committed herself to "a bit". All of them were extremely happy with the outcomes, in terms of their feelings about the day or residential placement, but they did not always associate this occurrence directly with the intervention of the care manager who had conducted their assessment.

Autonomy and building better family relationships

In three cases, the changes that had resulted from their assessment had given them a greater distance from their carer and family, even if this was just to go out to a day placement twice a week. Jane's position had not changed, but in fact she had stayed at home independently on her own for a week since the first interview, while her parents went to Scotland. Thus, all four had experienced relatively greater independence and autonomy than during the previous 12 months.

One of the questions we asked them was whether the assessment also 'helped things' for their carer, and all four of them gave much fuller answers than the first time, indicating their awareness of their carer's point of view:

> "My mum's going back to the [Elderly Persons'] Day Centre after Easter. It helps my mum for me to come here. She's going to get her pension today."

> "It's good for her that I'm coming here during the week."

Marilyn spoke at length about her mother, and her mother's feelings about her having left home. She felt that:

> "She does miss me, and she finds it so hard!... But it's better being independent, and I get on better with my mum now."

She then told the researcher about her efforts to provide presents and surprises for her mother, and was in fact planning a party for her birthday. These comments seemed to indicate what can happen for families when the individual with learning disabilities and the carer are not forced to live in such close proximity. In fact, another carer whose son had moved from home during the year told us of the more 'adult-to-adult' relationship which had developed between them.

These few examples certainly show that a separation of carer and cared for person, even on a part-time basis, can result in greater understanding and a better relationship between the two parties.

Friendship

All four of these people had happy tales to tell. For Jane, her week at home when she had managed on her own was a source of great pride. For Marilyn, her move to a new home had gone well. Fred was very enthusiastic about his work at the workshop, and loved showing the researcher the furniture he was making, and Julia particularly enjoyed the catering training she was receiving at the centre. She was hoping that this would eventually lead to employment.

Some common themes emerge from their experiences. One very positive factor for all of them were increased friendships and a better social life. Through the activities they were involved in, they had made contacts and friends, or renewed old friendships. Even Jane, who had merely stayed at home, had found that neighbours and friends got in touch during the week, and she was able to interact with them on her own. Fred had chosen to go to the woodwork centre partly because of a particular friend whom he knew there, but he now was not so dependent on this one friendship. He said:

> *"I've got other friends here now. I've got a new girlfriend."*

Conversely, he had stopped going for short breaks in a particular hostel, because of: "somebody there I could not stick".

Clearly, the opportunity to do new activities, or to live in a new way, was important as it opened up avenues for new social connections.

Choices of occupation

Marilyn had chosen to keep up her former voluntary work in a charity shop, and Jane's favourite (unpaid) work placement was her day a week doing office work in a local voluntary organisation. The two people who had started new day activities were involved in very different occupations: woodwork and catering.

The variety of these occupations shows the importance of choice. These four people had been given the opportunity to sample, or simply to see, some different options so that they were not forced to continue with a particular activity, simply because that is what they had done in the past. Julia, for example, had said at the time of the assessment that her favourite activity was 'sewing', since she had previously worked in a sheltered work situation, making cushions, for sale in the local market. Her placement was also imaginative, in that she was in a centre that was not defined by the label 'learning difficulty'. Clients there had a range of support needs, and many had physical impairments. What they had in common was their desire to benefit from the particular training on offer at that centre.

It will, however, be noted that all four of these people were doing work that was largely voluntary when they were re-interviewed, as were all the working individuals in the study. Fred was being paid a nominal sum of £8 a week for his two days' work, about which he was very enthusiastic. The government's Welfare to Work programme aims to allow as many disabled people to work as wish to. Advice and information on employment are often needed, but are not always available, and there are many disincentives for disabled people to take up paid work.

Independence

A fourth theme to emerge from the accounts of these four people was that of independence. All of them had found greater independence than they had enjoyed a year previously, and they were all very happy with the new opportunities this gave them. Jane said:

> *"I have been using a microwave quite a lot now, since mum was away, and I am doing my own shopping, getting the paper. Wednesdays I do the lottery."*

Since her week's independent living, she had kept up these new activities, and her weekly lottery ticket had even resulted in a prize of £75!

Marilyn said:

> *"It's brilliant. I have some choices [about food] and I can cook here."*

Their new found independence gave all four people an enhanced self respect, and they were all pleased to show me in some detail what they were doing, and how things had worked out for them.

Reviewing and monitoring the care plan

Although these four examples are among the very positive ones in our sample, none of them claimed to have seen their care manager more than once since starting the new activity. Jane had been referred to a social worker, in order to start thinking about future placements. She had only had one brief visit, resulting in the promise of further visits to housing options: these had not yet materialised. Marilyn's social worker had left, and she now had a new one whom she claimed she had "not seen much of", while Julia had not seen her social worker since her placement, and nor had Fred.

Doubtless the assessors involved felt that they could not keep making visits to placements once they were satisfactorily arranged, but some contact would be useful, even if it was arranged through a third party. All four of the individuals followed up here wished to see their care manager again, and would have liked to discuss options for the future. For all of them, the present arrangements were fine as far as they went, but were seen as a stepping stone to the future, rather than an end in themselves.

Jane, for instance, had become quite clear in her mind that she wished to live at home, and take over the house in her own right, if and when her parents died. Fred also was more assertive in talking about the future, and said he "might like to move in with a friend".

One change in a person's life can open the door to many more, and so people need someone to talk with, and to continue to make new arrangements and choices.

6

Sorting out conflicts of interest

Chapter summary

- Care managers and key workers are far more likely to perceive conflicts of interest than the families themselves. Carers tended to see disagreements as a normal part of family life.

- Professionals should be careful not to stereotype carers. They need to spend time to discover their real perceptions and feelings.

- There were sometimes disagreements in families when the carer needed a break, but the disabled person did not want to go for a particular short break. Instead of being persuaded to go, they should be offered more choices.

- People with learning disabilities, on the whole, were anxious not to upset the balance of the family situation.

- Disagreements where the carer was trying to persuade the cared for person to do something, particularly like a short-term break, tended to be resolved by professionals in favour of the carer.

- Disagreements which were about increasing independence skills tended to be resolved in favour of the person with learning disabilities.

- The Carers Act has not made a great deal of difference to the way in which conflicts are resolved. Good advocacy for both carer and the cared for person is the best way to deal with such conflicts.

Why look at conflicts of interest?

Many professionals are increasingly aware of the potential for problems arising from conflicts of interest within the family. The introduction of the formal carer's needs assessment has the potential to highlight this problem in that it gives formal recognition to the rights of the carer, beside those of the service user. We were particularly interested to follow up cases where a disagreement had arisen, and to see how it was resolved by all three parties. The question we put to the carer was: 'Was there any disagreement between yourself and X about the services your family needs?'

Table 5: Disagreements identified by

	Assessors	Carers	Individuals
No disagreement	20	32	39
Current disagreement	23	19	12
'Past' disagreement	5	–	–
Potential disagreement	3	–	–
Total number	**51**	**51**	**51**

As will be seen from the above table, assessors (care managers or keyworkers) are more likely than the families themselves to perceive disagreements. If potential and past disagreements are included, 61% of assessors believed families had experienced, or were likely to experience, a disagreement between carer and cared for person.

Assessors' views on conflicts

Why did this mismatch of perceptions occur? In some cases, what the assessor defined as a conflict of interest was simply not put in those terms by the carer. Parents, in particular, saw many differences of opinion as part of family life, and as something that would be sorted out naturally within any family. The fact that their son or daughter was 40 rather than 14 had no bearing on this. For instance, a daughter who refused to go to a short-break hostel was just another part of family life to the mother, while to the assessor, the situation was one of conflict. This accounted for eight cases in which the assessor saw a conflict of interest, but the carer saw none.

Many of the keyworkers and care managers had a very good understanding of the rights of the individual, and so most of the conflicts that were identified resulted from a genuine attempt to understand the viewpoint and needs of the individual, and to weigh these against those of the carer. For instance, people who worked with and knew an individual at his day placement could see that he preferred certain types of food, or certain activities, which on occasions conflicted with the cultural, religious, or other preferences of his family. These workers saw the individual's right to choose as more important than the family's right to appropriate cultural treatment.

There were seven other instances where the conflict spoken of by the assessor was in fact a different one from that spoken of by the carer. Carers tended to talk more about domestic arrangements, or the fact that their son/daughter did not want to do certain things when asked to help around the house. Assessors, on the other hand, were more likely to talk about the long-term interests of the disabled person than about domestic arguments.

There were three cases where the assessor appeared not to have had the time fully to explore the carer's real aspirations and feelings about a situation. It was easy for them to stereotype a family as 'worrying' or 'anxious' about independence or risk-taking. On the contrary, sometimes these parents seemed to be very proud of their son or daughter's wish for independence or achievement, and the situation was not as black-and-white as it appeared to the assessor.

All this, of course, underlines the need for more time and private discussion with carers, and training of staff in the avoidance of stereotyping.

Carers' views on disagreements

The most common disagreement that carers spoke of was where they needed a break but their son or daughter was reluctant to leave the family home and go to stay in a residential hostel. Five carers mentioned this situation. There were a few other individual differences, concerning moving out of home, and the right to establish relationships, including sexual relationships. There were also many relatively minor domestic arguments mentioned, relating to chores around the house.

These are all fairly predictable occurrences within families, and it ought to be stressed that the majority of people we spoke with lived in apparent harmony: 29 carers said there was no difference in view between them and their disabled relative:

> *"James is such an easy person to live with, and he loves his own home and privacy. I would be completely on my own without him – there isn't the loneliness when there's someone else in the house with you."*

Many parents, in particular, spoke of how they could 'read' their son or daughter's feelings, even with people who were non-verbal. They said they would know whether or not the person was happy about something.

There were also very many stories about ways of persuading someone to do something. People who did not want to try out the local hostel were gradually encouraged to do so by repeated visits to see the place or personal approaches from members of staff they knew well. As this mother put it:

> *"He pushes the boundaries – but I can get him round to my way of thinking."*

Such persuasion strategies were generally not available to the individuals with learning disabilities, and so their end of the arguments had to be fought either with the assistance of a member of staff at the day centre who spoke up for them, or by unexplained sudden refusals to go to clubs, day centres or hostels.

Parents and carers often expressed a clear commitment to respecting the individual's wishes, and were nearly always very proud and happy when their son or daughter developed the skills to speak up. One young woman had recently started using a communication device that enabled her to express her views, and had spoken up in student council meetings at her centre. Her mother was very happy about this, and was listening to her daughter's newly expressed wishes to try out a group living situation.

However, it is probably true to say that most parents were keener on decisions that suited them, and fitted in with their own best judgement. Many carers we spoke with did not take seriously their relative's ability to make decisions for themselves, and they saw their own role as smoothing over situations, so that they did not reach crisis point. "I have to sit and talk her out of things" was a very common theme. This related to the view that most parents had of their son or daughter as immature, or even still as a child. "She is 33 going on 12", as one mother put it. Another parent referred to her daughter as going through the "teenage rebellious stage" in her thirties.

The views of people with learning disabilities on disagreements

From the point of view of the individuals we talked with, there were few conflicts. Out of the 34 who could speak for themselves, 22 said that they and their parents/carers agreed about things, and that they both wanted the same things from the assessment. Only five really reported any disagreement, although in another seven cases some kind of conflict of interest could be inferred through other things they said.

Of these 12, four people talked about levels of independence: wanting to be more independent in some way (eg by doing tasks such as cooking, by going out more, or indeed by moving out of the parental home). Two had plans in motion to move on, and in both these cases, the parents had been consulted by day centre staff about the situation. In

both these cases, the parents did appreciate their son or daughter's viewpoint.

In five other cases, the disagreement was the other way – the parent/carer wanted at least some breaks, and wanted their relative to have residential breaks, or even to move into residential care. In almost all these cases, the parent had persuaded their son/ daughter to go for a break, often by a long process of gradual familiarisation, either with the actual place s/he was to go to, or just with the idea of going. One mother spoke of how they "talked it out", so that she could "make him see reason". Her son said:

"Yes, I'm going on this holiday, aren't I, to see what it's like."

Of course, carers often do have a real need for such a break if they are to continue caring at all, and several of the individuals realised that this was the reason they had to go to the hostel occasionally: to "give her a break". This issue may cause conflict to some extent, but they are hardly conflicts of interest: if the individual wishes to stay living at home, it is in his or her interest that his or her carer should have a break and be more able to carry on caring.

It is worth noting that three of the issues identified from people with learning disabilities had not been reported by either assessor or carer. Problems or aspirations were mentioned by individuals that had not been taken into account in the assessment at all. These included the wish to be more independent, to go out in the evening, and to have more rests from work at the day centre.

However, as in most parent–son/daughter relationships, the attitude of the individual towards his/her carer is *not* generally one of open conflict. As one person jokingly put it:

"We do agree – it's better than kicking her up the backside! When my mum kisses me, I wipe the kisses off."

This seems to sum up rather neatly the stance that many of these people took towards their carers. Wiping the kisses off, but remaining fundamentally dependent on their carers' wishes and dictates, this group of people were anxious not to upset the balance of their family situation.

Dealing with conflicts of interest

One person with a learning disability spoke of the dilemma for the social worker who worked with her family:

"She tries to be neutral, but she always ends up taking one of our sides."

How did keyworkers or care managers deal with situations in which they felt there was a genuine conflict of interest?

In the IPP, disagreements did not necessarily emerge during the actual meeting, but some meetings reflected those disagreements. For instance, one individual's wish to have a particular person at the meeting had been countered by his mother, and in this case the centre respected the mother's wishes. In another situation, the individual's wish to get paid employment had already been talked through with parents, and so a benefits advisor was invited to the IPP meeting, and was able to reassure the parents about benefits issues. Thus, in arranging the IPP, staff often had to do some pre-planning, and in general the aim of this planning seemed to be that disagreements should be dealt with beforehand, and not intrude on the actual meeting.

In the full care management situation, the assessor had formal opportunities to hear both sides of any conflict, and they often tried to do this. In particular, they nearly always saw the carer individually, without the person with a learning disability, and also saw the individual outside the family situation, often at a day centre. Problems, however, arose when no day placement existed, since it was impossible to find a place where the person with a learning disability would feel comfortable and want to talk. There were at least three people with learning disabilities who had not really had an independent assessment outside the family home.

Methods for dealing with conflicts of interest often amounted, in the end, to similar strategies to those used by parents to "smooth over the differences" or

use gentle persuasion. The difference was that the assessors could use gentle persuasion on carers, as well as on service users, and often did so.

"I listen to them both individually, and then I achieve a negotiated compromise."

The compromise achieved, of course, could favour the carer's or the individual's viewpoint. In practice, disputes where the carer was trying to persuade the individual to go for short-term breaks were resolved by assessors in the carer's favour, while disputes where the individual was anxious to become more independent were resolved in the individual's. Often sheer pragmatism dictated the outcome of these situations. As one assessor put it:

"It's a balance. It's weighing up the risk of it [short-term breaks] not happening. In order for X to stay at home, K has to have breaks from caring."

More than one assessor had talked with the carer, over a period of time, about issues relating to the individual moving on. They had also taken pains to help families become accustomed to the idea of more flexible day care provision, or more flexible short breaks provision. This was usually done on a one:one basis, and was a time-consuming process, involving a good deal of listening and discussion of views on both sides.

Has the Carers Act made a difference to conflicts of interest?

The conclusion is that the Carers Act has not made a great deal of difference to resolution of conflicts of interest, except in so far as the carer has an 'official' chance to state his/her side of any dispute. Social workers and keyworkers do see themselves primarily as advocates for the individual with learning disabilities, and legislation prior to the Carers Act (eg the NHS and Community Care Act) supports this situation.

However, where a carer needs a break and the individual does not want one, the importance of meeting a carer's needs generally has to predominate. Consequently, there are still some people with learning disabilities who are persuaded to go off for short breaks that they do not like. The message to social services departments and other organisations must be to develop a wider range of services, to give users more choice about the type of break they receive.

A good carer assessment is not about denying self-advocacy to the disabled person. It should go along with an approach that enables people with learning disabilities to speak up for themselves in whatever way they can, and to be listened to. Providing the person with learning disabilities with more information, and paying attention to their detailed wishes will resolve many potential conflicts of interest. The carer assessment, likewise, should enable the carer to consider him or herself as a person, with needs of their own. From the evidence in this study, an assessment does not increase the likelihood of conflicts of interest, but can help to resolve them.

Where there is a genuine and open difference in viewpoints, it is very hard for the same professional to listen to and advocate for both parties. The most radical and successful solution to this problem was for two different assessors to see the carer and the individual. In the family where this had happened, at least for the time being, a more balanced and open discussion had been fostered, and all parties appeared to be very happy with this at the time we saw them. As this mother said,

> *"I found it very helpful, because I was very frustrated with the former social worker.... Richard needs to be able to have somebody to stand up for what he wants, and somebody different to be able to stand up for my needs. There is a conflict between what Richard sees as OK and what I see as OK."*

One year later

Chapter summary

- **We re-interviewed 43 of the 51 carers after approximately one year, and found that their circumstances had changed quite dramatically in many cases. These changes seemed to be far more significant than the outcomes of carers' needs assessments.**

- **There had been many changes in families due to the increasing maturity, assertiveness, or in some cases, problems of the person with learning disabilities.**

- **Families at the 'transition to adulthood' stage were badly prepared.**

- **Several families reported an increase in the problems they faced, such as an additional family member becoming disabled.**

- **Carers had often suffered bouts of ill-health during the year.**

- **There was an increase in 'mutual caring' within some families.**

- **Services had changed during the year, partly due to cuts.**

- **Reviews of day services caused mixed reactions, but on the whole there was a demand for services that reacted flexibly to individual need.**

- **Any assessment of need must be continuous, to keep track of all these changes.**

Introduction

The assessment process should not be viewed as a 'one-off' event. As many practitioners pointed out, and as is reinforced by the government White Paper (DoH, 1998), assessment of need should ideally be viewed as a dialogue between the care manager, the service user and the carer, a continuous process of identifying needs and providing services.

The 51 families who took part in the second phase of the study were approached again after approximately one year, for follow-up interviews. A total of eight families were lost to the study: two were untraceable, and six declined to take part again, mainly because of lack of time, stress or ill-health. For further details of the methodology used, see Chapter 1.

All the follow-up visits were extremely relaxed and friendly, due to familiarity with the interviewer. There was a sense of pursuing a conversation we had started on the previous interview, and this did help carers and people with learning disabilities to be honest and open about their views.

Table 6: **Numbers of carers re-interviewed after one year**

	1st stage interviews	2nd stage interviews (one year later)
Carers Act assessments	20	18
IPP (Service Review)	25	22
Children Act assessments or ongoing	6	3
Total	**51**	**43**

Any assessment is only as good as the outcomes, and we were therefore keen to find out how our sample of families had fared after a gap of about one year, and how, in retrospect, they now viewed the carer assessment or other form of assessment they had received.

Other research, both before the Carers Act and since, has revealed the tensions which exist between needs-led and service-led assessment (Ellis, 1993; Baldwin, 1996; Davis et al, 1997). The White Paper *Caring for people* (DoH, 1993) states:

> *The objective of assessment is to determine the best available way to help the individual ... assessments should not focus only on the user's suitability for a particular existing service.* (DoH, 1993, p 18)

However, Baldwin (1996) finds the practice of care managers to be based on a "web of uncertainty" (p 54). Brammer (1997) reports on the effects of the Gloucestershire Case, where a series of High Court decisions were made relating to whether or not a local authority was under a legal obligation to meet the needs of disabled people, regardless of resources. The final stage of that story was the House of Lords ruling, which recognised that service-led assessment was the norm:

> *Needs for services cannot sensibly be assessed without some regard to the cost of providing them.* (Lord Nicholls of Birkenhead, quoted in Brammer, 1997, p 33)

The focus of this study has been carers, but as we found in the first part of the research, carers' interests are usually best served by provision of good quality and appropriate services to people with learning disabilities. Banks (1999) also argues for a widening of the concept of carer support, beyond "marginalised" carer services:

> *Carers say that the priority outcome for them is achieving a good quality of life for the person they care for.* (Banks, 1999, p 14)

Before turning to the issue of service outcomes, however, it was apparent that other changes had occurred in the circumstances of many of these families during the year, and these should be

mentioned first. They were often far more important than any outcome of the carer assessment.

Changes in family circumstances

Changes in the person with learning disabilities

Carers told us of many ways in which the person with learning disabilities they cared for had changed during the year. These were nearly always in the direction of growing assertiveness, or perceived maturity, and we were given several examples of people who were now more able to speak for themselves and make decisions. Carers and parents were proud of these achievements, and were happy that their son or daughter was 'growing up'. However, occasionally the changes had caused tensions and problems in the families.

With many of the younger people with learning disabilities, the family had become more aware of 'transition issues', and were now thinking quite differently about the future. One family, whose son was away at residential school for long periods, had been invited to a school review, and were shocked to find that the review was the first official 'transition' one, and they were being expected to make decisions about the future:

> *"At the school review we were asked, I mean they sort of dump this on you, 'Would you like him to stay at school?' And we sort of sat there with our mouths open ... nobody forewarned us that they were going to ask that question."*

Families who had already reached the next stage, beyond the boundary of 'age 18', found that they were not being supported in the same way as they had been during childhood. They felt in particular that their own role as parents or carers was undermined, since they were entirely unprepared to think of their son or daughter as an autonomous adult:

> *"Now she is an adult, there's other adults that take charge, and we are sort of left out in the cold a bit, I feel."*

Additional problems in the family

Although a year may seem like a short time, there had been several really important changes that affected the circumstances of the families we re-interviewed.

For instance, in two families an additional member had been diagnosed as disabled since the previous interview. This resulted in the original 'carer' now becoming a multiple carer. In reality, this process was, of course, gradual, but the actual diagnosis did have an effect on the family. One set of parent carers put it like this:

"I mean we have got two handicapped kids you might say ... and we are banging our heads against a brick wall with both of them."

In the second family, a grandchild of the 'carer' had been diagnosed as disabled during the intervening year, which had a knock-on effect on the whole family. The daughter who had previously given her mother support could no longer do so, and in fact the mother was now in the position of frequently having to provide childminding services for her other grandchild, while her daughter kept appointments. This was in addition to still being the main carer for her own son with learning disabilities.

The effect of having two people with support needs in the family was more than a simple addition of needs. This was largely due to the fact that there was no communication between the two sets of professionals who provided assessment and support for each disabled person. "The two things are separate", these parents said, leaving the carer(s) in the middle, with no one to consider their position in trying to meet two sets of needs. In one family, the additional diagnosis had meant that both parents had to be 'on duty' almost constantly, as one parent needed the back-up of the other at all times.

Eight carers in our study mentioned increased stress when we re-interviewed them after one year. In some cases, this had resulted in resignation and depression, as illustrated rather bleakly in this comment:

"I've got no ambitions now, all the hope I used to have is gone – it's just as we said, we are just living in limbo, from day to day."

Stress was caused by many factors, and was certainly not only due to the person with learning disabilities. More usually it was frustrations due to the support services and systems not working smoothly that caused carers to complain of crises. One carer said she had become very angry because of a breakdown in the support she was supposed to receive from a short-break service. She had taken out her stress on her son. Afterwards, of course, she felt so confused and guilty about the incident that this added to her existing problems.

Stress was sometimes held to be the cause of physical health problems that carers had developed. One mother felt that 'stress' was used as a simple explanation by medical practitioners, who took the easy way out by attributing everything to stress:

"I said, why have I got blood pressure? And he said 'stress of life'. I said, Oh God, it isn't the stress of life at all, they put it down to stress of life – why?"

Degeneration of carer's health

Despite the viewpoint expressed above, it was true that several of the carers in our sample had health problems which had become major obstacles by the time we met them again. Some of these were new, and others were escalations of previous problems, but all took their toll on the carer's ability to cope. Two of the carers we re-interviewed had developed major and devastating back problems, and another was awaiting a knee replacement. A fourth had been diagnosed as diabetic, affecting her ability to drive, and three others had suffered health crises which had resulted in hospitalisation. Such events, of course, impinge not only on the carer, but on the whole family, and the way in which they manage. When the carer is absent in hospital, solutions have to be found to care for the person with learning disabilities, and these can in turn have 'knock-on' effects.

The health of the carer and of the person with learning disabilities are closely intertwined, and episodes of ill-health experienced by one can easily affect the other. We were told of various illnesses suffered by the person with learning disabilities, including epilepsy, bronchial problems and scabies. All these had also had an effect on the carer's health and well-being. For instance, one man who had suffered bronchial problems was usually able to go for walks with his mother, to the local shops. However, due to his illness, he found any walking very difficult, which restricted not only his own mobility but also that of his mother, who found the wheelchair quite hard to manage.

Carers were reluctant to seek medical advice, and told us they avoided going to see their doctor "as a patient", presumably because they were so used to going with the person they cared for.

"I want to just keep working, and I can forget about everything else that is going on around me, and the fact that my health is not that good, but you know I will just carry on."

Their attitude was often one of 'ignore it and it will go away'. Carers tended always to put themselves in second place.

However, they were equally aware that any adverse outcome for them would have a catastrophic impact on the life of the person they cared for. Several carers spoke openly to us on the second interviews about the fear they had of dying, and leaving the person with learning disabilities without any firm plan or preparation for the future. As one elderly parent said:

"When I suddenly drop down dead, then something is going to have to happen."

This echoes what carers had said to us in the first phase of the project, relating to future plans. One of the greatest, still unfulfilled, needs for these families was planning, and preparing the individual for life beyond the family circle. Even those few who still felt quite fit and well were aware that future planning would be a wise move, since:

"Just because I don't have any needs now, doesn't mean to say I am not going to in the future, because I am getting older."

Increase in mutual caring in the family

A caring relationship is seldom a straightforward 'carer/cared for' situation, as we had already noted in the first part of our study. Frequently, the person with learning disabilities was taking on various care tasks in relation to their parent or 'carer', and we found that these had increased in the intervening period. Five families had now become aware of this situation, and of their mutual dependence within the family. One carer reported a conversation she had had with a member of staff at the day centre:

"I said the only thing that worries me, I said, that I will keep him home long enough that he will finish up caring for me, and she said 'What's wrong if that's what he wants to do?' and that's the first time anyone has said that to me."

The carer's increasing illness or frailty put them in a dilemma. It sometimes forced them to think of future residential options for the person with learning disabilities, but it could also have the effect of making them more dependent on that person, for both physical support and company. One elderly mother had suffered acute problems, necessitating an operation, followed by hospitalisation. She agreed that this made her aware she must plan for the future of her son, but she also said:

"If he went away now, it would mean living here on my own, which I don't really relish. Sometimes I don't know what I should do without him, sometimes I don't know what to do with him!"

This statement seems to summarise the impasse in which such carers found themselves. They badly needed to talk through these situations, and to find viable solutions which valued their own lives and needs. In fact, this situation was raised more than once at the mini conferences we ran. Parents who had spent a lifetime caring felt that their own lives were being "put on a scrap heap" and that they would be left in isolation to manage as best they could with increasing ill-health and loneliness. There is an urgent need for recognition of the contribution of these parents, as well as practical support for their own health problems, disabilities and social needs. Most wanted desperately to keep in touch with their son or daughter, and wished only to have a continuing role in their lives.

Changes in service provision

Not all the changes that carers told us about were due to their own changing circumstances. Many more, in fact, were the result of changed service provision, and, again, a lot seemed to have changed in a year.

Budgetary cuts and reallocation of finances

Many of the service changes they experienced appeared to the carers to be due to budgetary cuts, on the part of either the social services department, or the health service.

There had been changes in several of the short-break hostels, and while some of these were part of longer-term reviews of which families had been well aware, they nevertheless found them disruptive. One of the main causes of disruption was the possibility of new staff taking over a service, who were unfamiliar with the person with learning disabilities, and were not trusted by the carer.

One carer told us of an incident in which the staff at the hostel had not given appropriate medication to her son and despite the parent's protest on the first occasion that this happened, the mistake was repeated. Incidents such as this can lead to a lack of trust, which is common in any case with new staff and new service provision.

Several parents in such situations advocated strongly for a more flexible system, in which a detailed person-centred plan could accompany the person, taking the onus off the carer if things went wrong.

There were also other effects of service changes. In the case of short-break hostels, for example, the reallocation of beds had meant that emergency beds were no longer available to families. This was a real and obvious need for nearly all the families we met. Some of these changes appeared also to be due to the lack of coordination between health and social services, so that as health provision withdrew, social services were expected to take it over, but with

diminished budgets. Families whose relatives had previously used health-funded short breaks, for instance, were quite often left in difficult situations.

"There is a debate hanging over our heads about whether he's a health case, a hospital case or not. He's a borderline."

In fact, this family, whose son was awaiting assessment, felt quite adamantly that they did *not* want health provision, but this was simply due to their awareness of the poor quality of the services for short breaks in that particular authority. The fact remains that it is the most difficult and needy of individuals who tend to 'fall between the stools' of health and social services, and we found that in the intervening year, at least three more carers were being plagued by worries relating to health/social services funding.

Reviews of day services

The tug of war between health and social services was only one part of the pattern for these families. Local government reorganisation also had an effect. Even in cases where this reorganisation had taken place some years previously, three families in one particular area had just been told that they would no longer be able to use the provision which they and their relative were used to. The process of consultation with their 'new' local authority had just started when we re-interviewed, but they were still quite distrustful and confused about this, partly due to their general lack of trust about forthcoming changes in day centres.

As we found in the first stage of our interviews, all the local authorities in which we were working were undertaking reviews of their day services provision at the time of this study. When we re-visited families, these reviews had of course progressed slightly further, although none of the day centres involved had actually closed, and no one had lost their day centre place.

Nevertheless, the effect of the expected changes was quite perceptible, and several carers spoke to us of their concerns and worries about the future. Many of them felt that they were dependent on the day centre, since this enabled their relative with learning disabilities to have a separate life, outside the family home. They could not perceive of a viable alternative, particularly for those with greater levels of need. Their experience in the past had been that changes to services tended to happen without any real respect for their views, and so any rumours of change were met with distrust:

"We were told we were safe, and all the mums stopped petitioning, and worrying about the children's hostel, and then suddenly got a letter a year later, and you couldn't do anything about it. It just said we are closing, here's the date."

However, parents and carers did not all cling to the concept of a 'nine-to-five' day centre, as was apparent at the mini conferences we subsequently ran. The theme of day services was very prominent at these conferences, and the debate about alternatives to day centres was often quite productive. Some parents in fact felt that the fear of closures was caused by worries, due to lack of proper explanation.

"... they think staff will be wandering around the region with mobile phones – there's the terror – our son or daughter will be hanging around on a street corner waiting [for a member of staff]."

This carer, however, felt that changes were an opportunity to improve services. Rather than complaints about changes, a more frequent theme that emerged was about lack of flexibility in services. What parents and carers really objected to was the fact that their relative had to fit into the service, rather than the service fitting the individual. One mother commented about a sitting service:

"Why do they have to be labelled, really like a high disability? There should be somebody there that you could call on for an hour, or an hour and a half, or something like that. I think I would prefer to rely on friends, because friends know them."

Inflexibility resulted in an inability on the part of services to see the individual's personal needs, and attempt to meet those needs. Carers told us of:

- a special college which would only accept students for full-time residential provision, instead of more flexible weekday packages;

- a hostel for short breaks that put all the residents to bed at 8.00pm;

- a day centre that had to have its grounds serviced by the local council, while clients who could have benefited from meaningful employment were doing 'keep fit' in the hall.

In the main, families whose relative had never been at a day centre were quite adamant that they did *not* want that option, and therefore the day centre reviews and the possibility of new planning suited them well. Several of them wanted some kind of supported employment and continued education for their son or daughter, and those whose relatives had multiple needs were no different from the rest. They too valued inclusion in the community, and wished for services that actually supported the individual's aspirations. One such family had found a solution in a residential scheme that provided work activities. However, at the time of our re-interviews, most of the other families had not really achieved their goal, although one young person who was leaving college did subsequently obtain supported employment within a self-advocacy project.

A year is clearly a long while in the lives of these families. The changed circumstances we found in so many of our families pointed strongly to the need for continuous reassessment of needs, as indeed Department of Health guidance recommends. A one-off snapshot, as is often provided by a carer's needs assessment, quickly becomes outdated, and there was a real need for the assessor to keep in touch with the family, and to provide a continuous service.

8

Outcomes of carers' needs assessments

Chapter summary

- **There were very poor outcomes in terms of services provided. Only 18 of the 42 services that had been discussed in the carers' needs assessments had been provided after approximately one year.**

- **Just over half the carers re-interviewed felt that the carer's needs assessment had been of some use.**

- **The factors that were important to them were:**

  - **recognition of their viewpoint as a carer;**

  - **having services supplied as a result of the assessment;**

  - **an efficient response on the part of the care manager;**

  - **care manager who kept in touch;**

  - **real choice of services offered;**

  - **effective interagency working;**

  - **continuing carer support.**

- **There were many examples of assessments where these factors were not in evidence. Despite the balance of satisfaction and dissatisfaction expressed generally, some carers felt very strongly that their assessment had been of no value.**

Services provided

In the context of changes that had occurred in these families, the outcomes of a carer's needs assessment held one year previously did not necessarily figure large. However, after one year, it would be expected that most of the issues discussed at the carer's needs assessment would have been resolved, and appropriate services put in place.

This was not always the case. The 18 people we re-interviewed, who had previously received a carer's needs assessment, told us about a total of 42 services which had been offered at their assessments. The majority of these had still not been provided after one year, as the table below shows:

Table 7: Outcomes of services discussed at the time of the carer's needs assessment

Services provided after one year	18
Services not provided after one year	24

Examples of services that had been talked about, but had come to nothing, included:

- home care

- befriending service

- future options for residential care

- appropriate choice of day activities.

It was not always clear what had been promised and what had not. On occasions, the carer thought that a particular issue had been discussed, but it had not actually been written down on the care plan. In any case, the record systems were very unclear to both carer and researcher alike. Nonetheless, our conservative estimates of non-delivery of services must be cause for concern.

Ongoing assessments

The children's teams hardly ever offered carers' needs assessments to parents of disabled children, as they argued that they took the parents' needs into account on a daily basis. The assessment of the child's needs was part of a continuous involvement between professional and family. One result of this way of working was that it was very hard to find any kind of record of assessment of needs for any of these children, or indeed for the family. It is therefore difficult to judge whether a particular service had been offered, or was simply asked for. In any case, only three of these families took part in the follow-up phase, and they mentioned a total of six services that had recently been offered to them. Half of these, again, had still not been provided when we re-interviewed after one year.

Table 8: Outcomes of services that had been discussed a year previously during 'ongoing assessments'

Services provided after one year	2
Services not provided after one year	3
Need for service had changed	1

Carers' satisfaction with the assessment after one year

Of the carers we re-interviewed who had had a carer's needs assessment, just over half felt that the process had been useful for them:

Table 9: Carers satisfied with their carer's needs assessment after one year

Full carer assessment	10 (56%) satisfied	8 (44%) dissatisfied
Ongoing assessment	2 (66%) satisfied	1 (33%) dissatisfied

While satisfaction outweighed dissatisfaction, this study revealed a greater proportion of dissatisfaction than some other recent research (eg Holzhausen, 1997). The main reason for more negative responses

appears to be that the methodology in this study allowed us to ask carers for a considered response, in the light of actual outcomes of the assessment, rather than just for a simple reaction to the process.

Factors leading to satisfaction with carer's needs assessment
Recognition: 'somebody in your own right'

Interestingly, some parents/carers still felt positive about the process of the carer's needs assessment, even when they had not been well served in terms of outcomes. For instance, one set of parents who had multiple problems to cope with said:

> *"I would advise anyone to go for one, because it does make you feel as though you are somebody in your own right, you need to be bothered with."*

The act of recognising the carer 'in their own right', and listening to them, was of itself valuable.

Outcomes

As one would expect, carers were more likely to say that the carer's needs assessment had been useful if services they needed *had* been supplied. Of the 10 satisfied customers, seven of them were carers for whose family at least one service had been provided by the time we re-interviewed. The actual services that had been provided, following the assessment, were as shown in the following table:

Table 10: Services discussed at the carer's needs assessment, which had been provided one year later

Day care/activity	5
Transport	1
Move from home into residential care	2
Viewing residential options	1
Sexual counselling	1
Increases in short-break care	3
Home support with physical care	2
Holiday for whole family	1
Rehousing	1
Reflexology course for carers	1

However, not all these stories were entirely positive. One mother had had to fight to get the increase in short-break provision that she had been assessed as needing, and another had to make a special plea to her GP for a supporting letter to enable her to be rehoused. Occasionally, the service provided was not satisfactory, as was the case with the home support, which was not entirely reliable.

Eight carers said that they had not found their carer's needs assessment useful and, of these, five had more than one service 'promise' still outstanding when they were re-interviewed, and two had one service outstanding. In one case, the social worker had sent a letter some months after the carer's needs assessment, asking whether the family still wanted a befriending service. The family's circumstances had deteriorated greatly during that time, in that another sibling had been diagnosed as disabled, the mother's health was severely threatened, and there was every sign of extreme stress in the family generally. The mother had attempted to reach the social worker by telephone, but was unsuccessful as the social worker only worked part time. She then received a letter saying that this particular social worker was moving to another area, and that the family's name had been taken off the list for the befriending service, since they had not followed it up.

Parents and carers whose relative had the greatest, or most complex needs, frequently felt they had been badly let down by the process and the outcomes of their carer assessment. One mother, for instance, said:

> "Well it's really been a complete waste of time, hasn't it? I feel desperately sorry for other parents starting out with a disabled child, because I know they've got an uphill struggle – a long, long slog."

In the end, the main experience of many families was that they had to do all the pushing, even after the carer's needs assessment, in order to achieve any service support.

Response from care managers

Carers appreciated prompt, efficient responses from the care managers they dealt with, as one satisfied customer reported:

> "If she says she's going to do something, she will do it in two days – she's back to you. She doesn't keep you hanging around."

Waiting for a service certainly took the edge off their satisfaction! In two cases, for instance, day placements had taken about six months to arrange. This was fine in one case, since the family felt that they were in touch with the care manager, and that he was contacting them and actively making arrangements on their behalf. In the other case, however, the communication appeared to have broken down at one point, and the family was unsure whether anything was going to happen.

Contact with care managers

The way in which care management works sometimes militates against any longer-term contact between care managers and a particular family. Nevertheless, there were some care managers who had succeeded in maintaining contact, and in all cases this was greatly valued, as one carer commented:

> "... she is my main contact really, she is very good really, very good, you know if I ring her up, obviously if she's not there, I always leave a message and she rings back or the next day."

Those families who were satisfied with efficient service provision generally felt confident enough to pick up the telephone to the care manager when needed. It was those for whom "everything had gone dead" who did not feel they had a direct link with any source of support.

Certainly, during the period immediately following the carer's needs assessment, it was vital for contact to be maintained. Otherwise, carers could feel very let down by the process.

Real service choices

Instead of simply providing a service, some care managers had taken great pains to make sure the family had viewed all the possible services, and had a chance to make a real choice. This was invaluable, since satisfaction depends on both the individual with learning disabilities, and the carers, being happy with a particular service – whether this is a day activity, an arrangement for short breaks, or a befriender.

By contrast, the dominant impression that parents and carers had was that access to services was a matter of chance. This applied even to services that had been discussed or noted at the time of the carer's needs assessment so that, when they *were* obtained, one parent commented:

> *"I am very pleased, it's like winning the lottery, if you know what I mean."*

Another family had visited a residential home after meeting one of the residents at a birthday party, and an elderly single father had heard about residential options from his pub landlady, who also ran a private residential home. It was clearly valuable that these families had effective social networks, but there were obviously problems in the information flow to them from professionals. Carers need the correct information at the correct time, and it is hard to achieve this without continual updating.

Many of the stories that carers told us were about occasions on which they had had to take the initiative to pursue an option for a particular support service. Those who were successful in this respect had the impression that they had only won out because of keeping their ear close to the ground, meeting with networks of parents and families, and jumping in quickly at the right moment:

> *"Well, I kept pushing, the [local hostel] said 'well, we have got an extra bed', so I jumped quickly."*

Some parents and carers had been very vociferous about services they needed. The carer's needs assessment clearly was not enough for them to get the services they needed, and they had often had to take matters further:

> *"I wrote a letter to the Director of Social Services, and sent a copy to the MP. I said I needed more respite care, not less, and I had a social worker round with her team leader discussing it with me. What he basically said was, the louder you shout, the more you get."*

This strategy of shouting loudly worked for some families, but it must be remembered that there are many others who would not, or could not, make their voices heard.

Interagency working

However, care managers were not always so good at attempting to find solutions to the obstacles that arose. For instance, in more than one case, the person with learning disabilities had wished to attend college, but had been unable to because of lack of transport. Such examples show the value of a more strategic response, where different authorities and agencies are working together more effectively. Interestingly, the best example we had of joint working was where a carer support worker (who had carried out the assessment) persisted in her arrangements with the social work team until a positive outcome was achieved.

Although their needs had already been assessed, in a general sense, at the time of the original carer's needs assessment, the experience of these families was that there was often still a lot of 'red tape' and paperwork to be negotiated before anything was delivered. This was a major cause of anxiety to the families concerned, who felt that they had to put over the 'worst case' scenario in order to obtain what they needed. One family who evidently needed rehousing had only got their GP to write a supporting letter by describing the depression the mother was suffering, as a result of the multiple disabilities and illnesses in the family. Another parent put it like this:

> *"You've got to get assessed and get into these things before you can even see what is going to happen, because it just takes so long for somebody to decide on what they are going to do, and who's going to pay for it."*

We met one elderly single carer, who needed home help to get his son up in the morning, due to his own deteriorating health. Although his GP supported this application, it was returned unsigned from social services, apparently due to a misunderstanding. The parent took it no further, despairing that anything could ever happen easily.

Continuing carer support

The story does not stop when a service has been provided successfully. Carers whose relative had a service provided, be it day care or residential provision, still needed support themselves. Those whose son or daughter had moved from the family home needed sensitive support to deal with their feelings of guilt, their new role, and their need to keep in contact with their relative. Where this did not happen, a carer's changing needs could be completely overlooked. Where care managers do not feel that it is their role to support parents in this way, then an alternative way could be found, perhaps through carer centres.

One carer support officer who had carried out a carer's needs assessment had managed to keep in touch with the family, even when the person with learning disabilities had 'moved on'. She recognised that the parents' needs are often greatest at this point, when feelings of guilt and adjustment to new circumstances can take their toll. The mother told us:

"She always finds two minutes. I know she's at the end of the 'phone if I need her. She just keeps in touch."

9

Service reviews (IPPs): what can they offer the carer?

Chapter summary

- IPPs have the great advantage of being regular, available and understandable.

- IPPs are centred on the person with learning disabilities, and the carer's needs are sidelined. The carer needs one:one time, which in general s/he does not get at the IPP.

- Most IPPs were very accessible for the disabled person.

- About two thirds of service changes promised by an IPP had been achieved after one year.

- IPP goals did not generally deal with comprehensive service changes, but with smaller adjustments.

- Carer satisfaction with an IPP did not appear to depend on the achievement of goals.

- Carers appreciated the IPP because it gave them:
  - referrals to other professionals;
  - communication with the day service;
  - a professional exchange between them and the staff.

- However, there was a large unmet need for better sources of information.

- In terms of record keeping, the care management assessment has much to learn from that of the IPP.

- A carer focus could be incorporated into the IPP process.

Availability and regularity

The main positive strength offered by the IPP system was its availability and regularity in contrast to carers' needs assessments, which only a very few carers receive. The IPP review system was not only widely available and regular, but also understandable. The structure of the meeting, the feeding in of written reports, the review of the previous year's goals – all of these things made it easy for families and individuals to understand.

Focus on the carer

An IPP is an individual plan that focuses on the service user and his/her programme of activities. Most carers had commented during their first interviews that the IPP meeting was entirely centred on the needs and perspective of the person with learning disabilities. It is in fact planned like this, so it is not surprising that carers will mostly find themselves sidelined. As one mother put it:

"I don't think it's meant to include my needs really, I don't think they are ever discussed."

This does not mean that carers therefore discount the process. The reality for many of these families is that it was the only regular source of support and communication they were being offered by service providers or funders.

In the carer's needs assessment, on the other hand, carers could theoretically have one:one time devoted entirely to their needs, so that they could feel empowered to talk from their own viewpoint. Although assessments were not always like this, this undoubtedly contributed to the strength of a well-conducted carer's needs assessment.

Accessibility

Accessibility for the individual was also an important feature. Some IPPs seemed to have been far more accessible than others, but none of the full care management assessments were easy to understand. Accessibility can mean many things, to different people, but the following features need to be taken into account:

- starting from the individual's own viewpoint and experiences;

- enabling the individual to have a voice, perhaps by providing aids to memory and communication such as photographs, videos, symbols;

- giving the person with learning disabilities time to prepare;

- giving them time to consider different services and form an opinion.

It is worth emphasising that accessibility here did not exclude a focus on the carer. On the contrary, carers were happier when there was a thorough way of ensuring that their son or daughter really did have a voice.

Service provision through the IPP

The 22 carers we met who had been involved in IPPs mentioned a total of 40 'services' that had been offered through the IPP process. Of these, two thirds had been provided after one year, one third had not, and in one case the need had changed.

Table 11: Outcomes of services or service elements that were discussed at the IPP

Service provided after one year	26
Services not provided after one year	13
Need for service had changed	1

The IPP figures do look far better than those from the carers' needs assessments, and it will be recalled

that there were only 18 positive outcomes from carers' needs assessments, and 24 services that were still outstanding. However, it is fair to say that the nature and scope of the services under discussion did differ. A typical service package at an IPP would be:

- speech therapy assessment

- increased days at centre from three to four

- referral to clinical psychologist to advise on behaviour.

Occasionally, however, the IPP did result in a change in short-break provision, and there was quite an overlap with the full community care assessment in this respect.

Carers' satisfaction with the IPP after one year

When we re-interviewed carers, we asked them several different questions about their views on the IPP process.

- Did you feel the IPP was useful to your relative with learning disabilities?

- Did you feel the IPP was useful to you as a carer?

- Was it a good way of meeting your needs, as well as those of your relative?

'Satisfaction' was only considered positive when the carer answered positively to both the second and third questions. In fact, nearly two thirds said that they were happy about the usefulness of the IPP for themselves, while one third did not feel the IPP had any value for them.

Table 12: Satisfaction with IPP after one year

Carers who found the IPP had been useful for them	14 (64%)
Carers who did not find the IPP useful for them	8 (36%)
Total number of carers re-interviewed about the IPP	22

Similar questions about the carers' needs assessments had yielded a satisfaction rate of 10:8 (56%). Since the IPP process is designed to focus on the individual with learning disabilities, one would not expect carers to feel that it had been useful in meeting their own needs. It is surprising, therefore, that a slightly greater proportion of carers felt positively about the IPP than about the carer's needs assessment. However, their criteria for 'satisfaction' may well have been very different in these two cases.

What do carers expect from an IPP?

By contrast with carers' needs assessments, carer satisfaction levels with IPPs were not obviously linked with the number of services that had been sorted out as a result. Of the 14 who declared themselves satisfied with the IPP, seven had had at least one service (or element of a service) provided since, while seven had had nothing that arose from the IPP.

This seems to indicate that carers' expectations of the IPP process are different from their expectations of a carer's needs assessment. However, it is interesting to see what kinds of services had actually been provided as a result of an IPP, and these are shown in the following table:

Table 13: **Services that had been discussed at the IPP, and were sorted out one year later**

Changes to day activities programme	6
Changes within short-break hostel	3
Community nurse visit	2
College course	2
Speech therapy	2
Viewing residential options	1
Extra day at existing placement	1
Coordination of short-break provision	1
Visual impairment aids	1
Bathroom aid at home	1
Work placements	1
Support in altering medication	1
Health advice	1
Support in rehousing	1
Advice on behavioural management	1
Clinical psychologist referral	1
Counselling to individual	1

There is a different flavour to this list, compared with Table 10 (services that resulted from carers' needs assessments). IPPs are more likely to deal with the fine detail of service provision, particular ways of managing behavioural challenges, or

problems that have arisen with existing short-break arrangements. They are less likely to discuss major changes in the pattern of someone's life, and are far less likely to really take on the family perspective.

Some carers also felt that IPP promises could be so worded that an agreed service could turn out to be fairly worthless when it was delivered. For instance, one young man had on his record of assessment that he needed to go for more trips into the community. During the year this had been fulfilled, since he had, in fact, gone out on at least two trips. However, both of these had been by minibus, and had been on days when the weather did not permit him to leave the bus in his wheelchair. As he had a severe visual impairment, the value of these trips to him was somewhat questionable.

"Piling them into the bus and driving them round for an hour and a half is an easy way of containment! It is not seeing the community."

IPPs that resulted in referrals to other professionals

On occasions, IPPs did consider more far-reaching topics, and these often resulted in a referral to another professional. Those who were most likely to be 'brought in' were members of a Community Learning Disabilities Team (CLDT), or similar.

In one family the individual with learning disabilities wished to move out from the family home, and in this case the IPP resulted in a referral for a full community care assessment. A chain of events was set off, including a carer's needs assessment, in which all the participants continued to work together. The keyworker who had referred the family continued to talk with the individual, to check on the parents' wishes, and to be involved in the practical visits to view residential provision. The mother commented:

"The last few IPPs we have had, we have achieved something, because they've said – oh, we'll do this and we'll do that, and they are doing it now."

From the carers' point of view, it was to be hoped that the IPP would be a vehicle to pick up any warning signals from them, and to refer the family on to a care manager so that the carer could receive a proper assessment.

Communication with the day service

Another positive function of their IPP, from the carers' point of view, was that it had kept them in touch with the life of their relative at the day placement. It helped them particularly to know the detail of what happened during the day, to talk about any problems day centre staff were facing, and to compare these with issues at home.

Families need to communicate with the day centre, or with any service which is providing for their relative. This applies equally well to schools and to school reviews. It is a way of formalising the contact between carer and institution, so that at least once a year there is an attempt to summarise the main issues.

The IPP as a chance for a 'professional' exchange between parents and staff

Six carers were happy the IPP had given them an opportunity to collaborate with the staff who cared for their son or daughter during the day. In this sense, the IPP became like a meeting of professionals, with the carer being accepted as a co-professional. This was particularly so with people with learning disabilities who could not speak for themselves, or who presented behavioural challenges. The parents/carers had found that the meeting was a chance to compare ways of managing problematic behaviour and to reach agreements.

"They have actually listened to the way I deal with him, and we see if we can't do a compromise of their way and my way and sort of meet in the middle."

Starting off a train of thought

Apart from the specific referrals that resulted sometimes from IPPs, carers also said that it had

sometimes helped in starting them thinking. This applied particularly where issues about future residential options, or about work, were raised. Sometimes parents/carers felt particularly worried about developments that might present risks to their relative with learning disabilities, and they urgently needed to air their views and to discuss the issues.

"It helped me to think about the future."

Information giving

There was a great and unfilled need for carers to have access to accurate, up-to-date and concrete information about what services were available. On the whole, care managers were more likely to have this information than keyworkers in day centres, but even care managers, as we have seen, were not always successful in this respect.

Record keeping in IPPs and carers' needs assessments

From the point of view of the person with learning disabilities, it is most important that the record of assessment can be understood and used. Care plans generally were not presented in such a way that they could be readily understood. Records of IPPs, however, tended to follow a distinct format for each centre or institution, which meant that they had the great advantage of being understandable and recognisable for families, as well as for the person with learning disabilities. They were seldom lost, and on the whole they were seen as meaningful.

Records of carers' needs assessments, where they were obtainable, had the potential advantage that they could be incorporated into the care plan for the individual. However, the record was often very brief indeed: in one case, the care manager had left the form with the carer to fill in, and this was done without any individual detail at all. Carers afterwards did not know if there was any record of the meeting they had had, nor did they grasp its possible significance.

Having asked the carers what they thought of their records, we then, with their written permission, examined records of assessments carried out for the interview sample. We were only able to obtain seven that related to community care plans and associated carers' needs assessments; all the remainder referred to IPPs.

The limited number of carer's needs assessment records can partially be accounted for by the inclusion of six children whose families were assessed under the 1989 Children Act. In these cases, assessments were often regarded by social workers as 'ongoing' and not suitable for separate carers' needs assessments because the families' needs as a whole had to be taken into account. Four records of carers' needs assessments were not received, although we know that they had taken place. This perhaps reflects social workers' general anxiety about carer's needs assessments, and having their work 'scrutinised'.

Carers' needs assessments

Of the seven sets of records received, one had been completed by the carer. As one would expect, the carer's needs assessments usually gave a full account of the tasks undertaken by the carer and their relationship with the person with learning difficulties. However, not all factors likely to impact on the caring role were covered. Few assessments mentioned the housing situation, any of the carer's outside work or caring commitments or the role of other family members in supporting the individual.

Equally, there was rarely a clear account of what plans had been made to meet carers' needs. For example, one parent expressed a need for both her son and herself to be provided with a holiday, more residential short-term care and some form of meaningful daytime activity. The social worker had summarised the services needed, but left blank the section about outcomes. Why this omission had occurred was not clear. Perhaps a lack of appropriate provision had prevented him from committing any clear plans to paper but without measurable objectives, there seems to be little point in going through the process of an assessment. It may protect the local authority from any risk of litigation for failure to provide services assessed as necessary, but it leaves the carer with limited scope for protesting.

IPP records

By contrast with the limited number of carer's needs assessment forms, we obtained copies of 22 of the 24 IPPs carried out among the interview sample. These records were generally very structured and the process was, as the name suggests it should be, client-centred. However, 10 of the IPP forms referred explicitly to the primary carer's need for services, and recorded those needs. Needs for certain services were cited especially frequently:

- residential short-term care
- home help
- financial support
- help with physical care in the home or overnight supervision at home
- more day care.

Sixty-six per cent of the interview sample were already using residential short-term provision and most requests by carers were for an increase in either the frequency or duration of breaks. In a few cases, families wanted more inhouse provision in order to prevent their son or daughter having to go so frequently to a residential service which they did not think suitable. In two cases, parents said they found that absence from home overnight tended to be associated with disruptive behaviour on their son's or daughter's return and this was a clear disincentive to using the residential provision which existed.

Where home help was needed, it was not generally requested in isolation but alongside day care or short-term care. Home help was often seen by carers as a means of 'keeping on top' of household tasks, including laundry, which could not be undertaken easily while the person with learning difficulties was at home.

All the people who had had an IPP assessment, were already using a day centre, although less than half did so on a full-time basis ($n = 10$). For those who had day activities on a part-time basis (including activities outside a centre), virtually all parents said they wanted a fuller programme for their son or daughter.

The IPP forms were often very specific about the goals and actions to be achieved in the coming year.

More often than not, these related to personal goals for the individual. For example, "to develop H's daily living skills" or "to ensure P visits dentist every six months". Sometimes the goals set involved carers taking an active role in reaching these targets and thus added to the carer's sense of responsibility:

"Mrs G to develop a scrapbook for M to use at home to keep him occupied."

Most goals set during IPPs were clear and measurable. Although most related to individual achievement, where there was reference to the delivery of services for carers, these too tended to be more specific, with a clear action plan and named worker assigned to the task. These are just some examples:

"... to establish regular respite Monday or Thursday nights and one weekend a month – residential social worker to organise."

"... to provide an extra day at day centre, specialist social worker and assistant manager of day centre to arrange with Mrs T."

In only two cases where carers' needs were identified was there a lack of such explicit plans. In one case, the carer's need for a break seemed to have been ignored completely when the action plan was written and in the other, while the same request was documented, it was not at all clear who was expected to make the appropriate arrangements.

From the documents analysed, therefore, it seems that carers' needs were often both identified and formally recorded through IPPs in ways that led to action.

The IPP in perspective

The kind of support being offered by day centres varied widely. In some cases, carers felt that they could always drop in, or telephone someone at the centre (usually a designated deputy manager or manager). Thus there was a known point of contact, and some centres were fulfilling the dual function of supporting clients and carers.

There is clearly a need for some kind of support and needs identification to be available to carers, other than simply for the few who can access carers' needs assessments. One possibility would be to use the vehicle of the IPP. A separate 'carer strand' could perhaps operate alongside the IPP, which could involve a visit to the carer, in order to talk about his/her own needs and views, in much the same way as the carer's needs assessment does. Then these needs could be taken into account during the IPP process, without intruding or detracting from the focus on the person with learning disabilities.

10

Conclusions and recommendations

Beyond the Carers Act

The main finding of this study was that the Carers Act is not working very well for the majority of carers of people with learning disabilities. It is only a small minority who are receiving any sort of carer's needs assessment, usually at a point of transition or crisis, and those who do receive them still have long delays in waiting for appropriate services. Therefore local authorities need to go back to the original spirit of the Carers Act, which was to assess carers' needs as a matter of course, so that crises and problems are prevented.

There were some good examples of successful outcomes from carers' needs assessments, and this study would want to endorse the value of a properly conducted carer's needs assessment. Where the care manager gave private time to the carer, and really listened to the range of issues and needs s/he had, and acted on the information promptly and efficiently, then a carer's needs assessment could be very valuable.

However, so many families are caring for someone with a learning disability who is not in active care management, and so the essential trigger for a carer's needs assessment is not happening. Social work teams are only able to prioritise those with urgent needs, or for whom circumstances have changed, and the Children's Teams we met do not routinely offer a separate carer's needs assessment. Therefore the majority of these families carry on from year to year without any direct contact with a social services team. The Carers Act should be seen as only one part of a much wider system to support these families.

The role of carer support officers

In this report, we have attempted to outline the perspective and opinion of each party to the assessment – the carer, the individual being cared for and the assessor. Where problems have arisen in identifying needs, the common theme seems to be a failure of communication, either for the carer or for the person with learning disabilities. As several assessors commented, some way has to be found for both carer and individual to have a separate, independent voice, and to have an advocate who is there just to listen to them.

In some cases, a carer support officer who is independent of service provision and budgets may be a good solution. Carers' centres at present often have problems in attracting and meeting the needs of carers of people with learning disabilities, who perhaps feel they have not got much in common with carers of elderly people or those with physical impairments. Therefore any attempt to provide independent carer support will probably need to be specific to this group.

All the families we met were asking for a better system of continuous support. Many saw the main service gap as being a need for professional, expert help. Carers are doing a really demanding job in supporting a person with learning disabilities in the family home, and they need not only to be accepted as co-professionals, but to receive the necessary advice, guidance and support that any professional would need. Carer support to this group of carers is not just about listening to them, or providing an advocacy service. It is about actually helping them with the job they are doing as carers.

These carers did not generally participate in carer support groups, or centres, and they would need to be assured of the value to them of any such service. However, a carer support service that was closely linked with the Learning Disability local services (day services, short-break hostels, supported employment, etc) would be far more relevant to them. With the changes that are being discussed to day services for people with learning disabilities, the needs of their family carers will have to be given serious consideration and planning.

Therefore the key recommendation here would be for local authorities to ensure that carer centres and carer officers are available. In some cases they should be enabled to carry out the carer's needs assessment. Where carer officers do deliver assessments, however, this should not result in letting care managers 'off the hook' with respect to their duties to consider the carer's needs. The primary role of a carer centre, as Fruin (1998) underlines, is "to provide information, emotional and practical support" (Fruin, 1998, p 19). If carer support officers are to deliver assessments, their role must be understood by all, so that their authority to identify needs and suggest resources is respected by budget holders.

Carer support and assessment of carer's needs through day services

This study saw that during one year the needs and circumstances of families can radically change. This means that there is a need to keep in contact, and to provide a service that continually monitors the detail of the family's changing needs. Most carers also wanted a more secure way of planning for the future, so that an individual's and family's wishes for future residential care were recorded, regularly updated and acted on.

The fact remains that social workers are for the few, while the majority of people access some kind of day service, although this may not be a bricks-and-mortar day centre. With the introduction of the care manager's role, the former ability of a social worker to offer long-term support to a family has been curtailed. This is seen as a dilemma by many

practitioners, and is still not properly understood by families themselves. However, practical solutions have to be found to meet the ongoing support needs of carers and families who do not now have day-to-day contact with the social services department.

A system already exists for most adults with learning disabilities, providing them with an individual review every year. This is referred to in most areas as an Individual Programme Plan (IPP). The system is geared entirely to the needs and wishes of the individual with learning disabilities, and it would be wrong to change that focus so that carers dominated. However, it might be possible to add an element of assessment of the carer's needs to the process, by providing the carer with a private opportunity to discuss his/her own needs and views, perhaps before the main meeting.

Day centres have to a greater or lesser extent taken on the role of providing support and information to families, and some keyworkers commented that families seemed to expect them now to be in a central, coordinating position in relation to services. One keyworker suggested that someone could be designated within the day centre, with time allocated to the role, in order to give proper information and advice to families.

Furthermore, day services are being reviewed in most areas, so that daytime opportunities can be more flexible. The issue of carer support therefore becomes even more vital. If these day services are expected to help families plan for the future and access services, authorities should consider some of the following:

- **a designated role of carer support officer within each day centre or day service, who could ensure that all staff know of their responsibility to involve, inform and support carers;**
- **a policy of seeing all carers personally in their own home, if possible, for a discussion that would be similar to a carer's needs assessment;**
- **staff training (perhaps provided by carers) in carer issues;**
- **an information and advice service within day centres or other forms of day service.**

These measures are likely to be especially important during the current period of reorganisation within day services, when families may lose the only reliable source of support they have.

Assessing the needs of people with learning disabilities

The above recommendations for day services in relation to carers should of course not be at the expense of the clients themselves. It should be reiterated here that some areas have developed excellent practice relating to clients' IPPs. It will be even more necessary to ensure that this good practice is spread if day services are to become more individualised and flexible.

- **People with a learning disability should have:**
  - **a designated keyworker, acting in many respects as an advocate;**
  - **a right to a one:one discussion prior to their IPP meeting;**
  - **staff who are trained in disability rights issues;**
  - **accessible information and communication strategies.**

Information and support for people with learning disabilities who take on caring tasks

As time goes on, people with learning disabilities are living at home with carers who age and may have disabilities or physical problems of their own. This study found a good deal of 'mutual caring' within such families. Although the parent/carer always felt that they were the carer, largely because of the responsibility they had to take on, we found many families in which the person with learning disabilities was providing both physical and emotional support for their 'carer'. This reveals a major gap in policy and practice.

- **Carers with learning disabilities should receive:**
  - **an assessment of their needs as carers;**
  - **formal support;**

- **appropriate training.**
- **More research and development should be carried out into this issue.**

Inter-agency coordination

As has been stressed throughout this report, families that include someone with a learning disability may have very many, complex and diverse needs.

The carers themselves may have impairments or other health problems, and there may be more than one person cared for. In addition, many of the people with learning disabilities have very complex needs. In all these cases, the number of significant professionals involved can be very high.

The suggested solution here was that statutory agencies need to see the carers themselves as equal partners, and, it should be added, the individuals with learning disabilities too. A round table discussion that brings together all the professionals involved with an individual was recommended. Of course, the IPP can often fulfil this role, if outside professionals are invited to the meeting. The possibility of holding this meeting in a place other than the day centre itself should also be considered, although the advantages of familiarity might outweigh the advantages of neutrality.

- **In addition to separate private meetings for carer and the individual with learning disabilities, there should be provision for a round table discussion with the individual, the carer and all the professionals involved.**

Staff training

As we showed in Chapter 4 in particular, there was considerable confusion among carers about the purpose of a carer's needs assessment. There was also much variation between teams, especially Children's Teams, in the way they assessed carers' and parents' needs, and this lack of clarity seemed to be reflected in the families' own perception of carers' needs assessments.

- Local authorities should:
  - clarify for all relevant staff who is entitled to a carer's needs assessment, and how they intend to deliver this commitment;
  - ensure that all relevant staff, including those who work with disabled children, understand the purpose of the carer's needs assessment and what it implies;
  - involve carers of people with learning disabilities in staff training;
  - involve people with learning disabilities (self-advocates) in staff training about disability equality issues;
  - ensure that the person delivering a carer's needs assessment can make clear to the carer the purpose and import of what is happening;
  - plan a strategy to enable people with learning disabilities themselves to access carers' needs assessments, when they start to take on caring roles.

Information about carers' needs assessments

We found that very few carers of people with learning disabilities had accessed any formal information about carers' needs assessments. As a group, they were largely unaware of their rights.

Once authorities are clearer about their own practice and intentions, an information strategy should be put in place, so that all families caring for someone with a learning disability know of their rights.

- Authorities should develop and regularly monitor a strategy for providing information to carers of people with learning disabilities, including:
  - information points at day centres and other day services, for carers as well as for people with learning disabilities;
  - newsletters distributed directly to families;
  - leaflets;
  - talks and discussion at carer centres and carer groups.

Record keeping

This is another area that our study showed to be very patchy. On the whole, it will be recalled, IPP recording systems had developed greater clarity and conciseness, together with more definite targets and goals, while carers' needs assessments themselves, and their incorporation into care plans, were very variable. In addition, the families themselves very seldom had a copy of their carer's needs assessment or care plan, and so were largely unaware of the potential force of these documents.

- Local authorities should review their record keeping systems for carers' needs assessments, taking into account the following factors:
  - records should be seen as an aid to the carer's needs assessment process;
  - forms for recording carer needs should be developed in conjunction with representative groups of carers, as some authorities have already done;
  - records should be concise and clear: they should be readable for carers and families, and also produced in an accessible format, so that the people with learning disabilities can understand their own assessment;
  - records should be quick to complete, and preferably in a uniform format so that everyone (families and assessors) understand records when they move from one system to another, for example from children's to adults' services;
  - records should be available to all parties concerned, especially the carer and the person with learning disabilities.

Planning for the future

A large number of families in this study were extremely anxious and uncertain about future plans for their disabled family member. This concern often clouded their life together, and their attitude towards caring. Solutions are desperately needed to address this situation.

Many parents spoke of the need for definite information about future plans for their son or daughter, because they have seldom been given any clear information about processes, timing and decision making arrangements for the future. Professionals may interpret these questions as a demand for security, but having a knowledge and understanding about procedures means that parents do not need to 'cling to' set plans.

At certain key points in the individual's life, this need for future planning becomes critical. These points certainly include the transition from children's services to adult services, the point at which the individual may be developmentally ready to live more independently, or the point at which the carer is becoming less able to provide care.

In order to avoid crises at these points:

- **there should be a coordinated and continuous service response to the family, that:**
  - ‣ **includes both the carer and the person with learning disabilities;**
  - ‣ **gives clear, concrete information about life-styles and future options, for example by direct visits to residential options, employment and leisure pursuits, and by written information, access to newsletters and data banks;**
  - ‣ **provides the family with role models for the future, for example by meeting people with learning disabilities, including self-advocates, who are living more independently;**
  - ‣ **gives a positive and clear message that the person with learning disabilities has rights to appropriate support outside the family situation;**
  - ‣ **records the wishes, of both the carer and the individual, at regular intervals, so that a life plan is gradually developed, that can be built on and altered as circumstances change.**

It is important that future planning is stressed in the government's agenda on carers.

New directions

The implementation of the Carers Act comes at the same time as several new directions in services for people with learning disabilities, which present both challenges and opportunities for carer support. The Direct Payments Act (1996) and the Disability Discrimination Act (1996) include people with learning disabilities in their provisions, underlining their rights to access ordinary community services and to decide for themselves what support they may need.

Although this study was not specifically examining the impact of service changes, there were day service reviews being carried out in most areas in which we worked. Some authorities had already developed, and others were developing, new and more flexible individualised services for people with learning disabilities. In one area in particular, this included an attempt to move in the direction of non impairment-specific services, so that people with learning disabilities might receive their support alongside other people needing extra support to live in the community. In the important area of short-term breaks, most authorities were making attempts to move away from residential hostels towards a more flexible service that would include family links. Family links were already very popular in children's services in all the authorities we visited.

Based as they are on beliefs in human rights and self-advocacy, these new directions nevertheless present challenges to families and carers. If their relative, for instance, no longer attends a day centre, but goes to a supported employment placement two days a week, and to a college course during term time, this may leave the carer both with additional 'on duty' time and with the loss of the support they previously received from the day centre.

Many carers in this study expressed worries about these developments, particularly in relation to day centres, since no clear plans had been put in place to ensure that family support would be ongoing. It is hard for carers not to be cynical about service changes, when their past experience has been that changes mean cuts. For instance, one family whose son has profound and multiple impairments was very anxious about day centre changes, which they felt would mean a loss of social contact and activity for their son when the 'more able' people left the day centre to move into community-based activities. Other carers expressed doubts about the value of self-advocacy, when individuals were not given real choices. They saw service providers as encouraging their son or daughter to have ambitions that were unrealistic.

It is particularly important at times of change and development to include the carers' perspective: it must be remembered that community services and support for people with learning disabilities were in many cases originally introduced through campaigning and pioneering work by parents and their organisations. Therefore, developments in philosophy and in service provision should never be imposed 'top down'. Consultation with carers should happen alongside consultation with service users.

- **Local authorities should:**
  - **include representatives of both carers and people with learning disabilities in the process of staff selection, at both service provision and local authority level;**
  - **consult with carers' groups when there is a definite task for them, and when they have the opportunity to make an informed contribution;**
  - **see interested families as a resource, and help them to contribute to local plans: individual carers may have the skills to suggest innovations in service provision;**
  - **find ways for self-advocacy groups and carers' groups to come together, so that they can share perspectives and ideas;**
  - **encourage peer support projects, where a more experienced disabled person meets up with a young person with a learning disability, which may help families to see their disabled member more positively, and provide opportunities for pursuing new activities.**

Finally, carers will rightly be cynical about new developments that encourage independence for their relative, if the reality is that these developments depend on *family* support. There is no substitute for additional resources to provide proper community support to people with learning disabilities.

If carers' needs are to be properly assessed and met, it is important that resources are both available and usefully directed. It is to be hoped that this study will help to re-direct those resources that are available, so that the needs of both carers and people with learning disabilities can be addressed.

As many carers in this study reiterated:

"If the services were right for him, I'd have no needs."

References

Baldwin, M. (1996) 'Is assessment working? Policy and practice in care management', *Practice*, vol 8, no 4, pp 53-9.

Banks, P. (1999) *Carer support: Time for a change of direction?*, London: King's Fund.

Beresford, B. (1995) *Expert opinions: A national survey of parents caring for a severely disabled child*, Bristol: The Policy Press.

Brammer, A. (1997) 'Community care assessment after Gloucestershire', *Tizard Learning Disability Review*, vol 2, no 4, pp 32-4.

CNA (Carers National Association) (1994 and 1995) Leaflet on research surveys, London: CNA.

Davis, A., Ellis, K. and Rummery, K. (1997) *Access to assessment: Perspectives of practitioners, disabled people and carers*, Bristol: The Policy Press.

Dobson, R. (1995) 'Fairer to carers', *Community Care*, June, pp 15-21.

Department of Health (DoH) (1993) *Caring for people*, London: The Stationery Office.

DoH (1995) *Carers (Recognition and Services) Act 1995: Policy guidance*, London: The Stationery Office.

DoH (1998) *Modernising social services*, White Paper, London: The Stationery Office.

DoH (1999) *Caring about carers: A national strategy for carers*, London: The Stationery Office.

Ellis, K. (1993) *Squaring the circle*, York: Joseph Rowntree Foundation.

Fruin, D. (1998) *A matter of chance for carers? Inspection of local authority support for carers*, London: DoH.

Grant, G. and Nolan, M. (1993) 'Informal carers: sources and concomitants of satisfaction', *Health and Social Care*, vol 1, pp 147-59.

Grant, G. and Whittell, B. (1999) *Family care of people with learning disabilities: Support for family coping*, Final report to NHS Wales, Office of Research and Development.

Holzhausen, E. (1997) *Still battling? The Carers Act one year on*, London: CNA.

Morris (1993) *Independent lives*, Basingstoke: Macmillan.

Morris, J. (1994) 'Prejudice', in S. French (ed) *On equal terms*, London: Heinemann Publishers.

Morris (1998) *Still missing?*, York: Joseph Rowntree Foundation.

NHS Executive (1998) *Signposts for success in commissioning and providing health services for people with learning disabilities*, London: DoH.

Nolan, M., Grant, G., Caldock, K. and Keady, J. (1994) *A framework for assessing the needs of family carers: A multi-disciplinary guide*, London: Rapport.

Nolan, M., Grant, G. and Keady, J. (1996)
*Understanding family care: A multidimensional model
of caring and coping*, Buckingham: Open
University Press.

Parker, G. (1994) *Where next for research on carers?*,
Leicester: Nuffield Community Care Studies
Unit, Leicester University.

Richardson, A. and Ritchie, J. (1989) *Letting go*,
Buckingham: Open University Press.

Robinson, C. and Williams, V. (1997) *View from the
top*, Report on the first stage of a research project
about the Carers Act of 1995, Bristol: Norah Fry
Research Centre, University of Bristol.

Shearn, J. and Todd, S. (1997) 'Parental work: an
account of the day to day activities of parents of
adults with learning disabilities', *Journal of
Intellectual Disability Research*, vol 41, no 4,
pp 285-301.

Todd, S. and Shearn, J. (1996) 'Struggles with time:
the careers of parents with adult sons and
daughters with learning disabilities', *Disability &
Society*, vol 11, no 3, pp 379-401.

Twigg, J. and Atkin, K. (1994) *Carers perceived*, Milton
Keynes: Open University Press.

Walmsley, J. (1993) 'Contradictions in caring:
reciprocity and interdependence', *Disability,
Handicap and Society*, vol 8, no 2, pp 129-43.

Walmsley, J. (1996) 'Doing what Mum wants me to',
Journal of Applied Research in Intellectual Disabilities,
vol 9, no 4, pp 324-41.

Williams, V. and Robinson, C. (1998) *A seamless
service?*, Bristol: Norah Fry Research Centre,
University of Bristol.

Winmax (1998) *Scolari*, London: Sage Publications
Ltd.

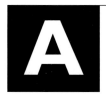

Appendix A: Methodology

The initial aims of *In their own right* required us to make contact with carers of people with learning disabilities who had recently received an assessment of their needs.

In each of the five areas in the study, we worked with the Social Work Teams or Community Learning Disability Team (CLDT) responsible for care management for adults with learning disabilities, and we also approached Children's Teams. The aim was for these professionals to pass on information about the project to families to whom they were offering a carer's needs assessment, who could then decide whether or not they wished to participate, and contact us directly. We hoped to find 100 families to interview, over the five authorities, in the course of about 10 months. Interviews with carers were semi-structured conversations based on a schedule of questions, and encouraging discussion of issues that were important to the people themselves.

Low number of carers' needs assessments

During the pilot stage of the project, we found great difficulties in reaching families and gaining consent to conduct interviews. This was due to a number of factors:

- there were clearly not many formal carers' needs assessments taking place;

- social workers and other professionals were unsure and unclear about carers' needs assessments, and perhaps felt that their practice needed to be 'tightened up' before they could take part in a research project;

- families themselves were unclear about whether or not they had received a carer's needs assessment, as was apparent from other research (Holzhausen, 1997);

- even when all these hurdles had been successfully negotiated, a carer might still not wish to take part in the project, perhaps because of overwork and stress, or perhaps through cynicism about the services or research.

In the five authorities, the ways in which carers' needs assessments were carried out were very varied. For example, some authorities, due to lack of resources, were restricting the offer of an assessment to families where there was an imminent change of service provision on the horizon. Other authorities passed on some carers' needs assessments to a carers' specialist organisation. Even within authorities, there were many different models, resulting in formal or informal assessments.

What was evident was that the families receiving a carer's needs assessment represented the tip of the iceberg. They appeared to be families for whom there were extreme changes, caused either internally (eg by death or illness) or externally (by service changes). The vast majority of families where there was someone with a learning disability were more likely to be receiving regular services, in particular day care services, which nearly all provide a service review (or IPP as they are often called).

While the service review was focused on the service user, and his/her needs, these reviews varied in the extent to which they involved the carer in the process, the way in which they were structured, and the extent to which the carer's needs were considered.

Broadening the research focus

We therefore decided to broaden the focus of our project, in order to reflect what was actually happening for carers, and to compare different kinds of assessment process and their impact on the carer. The changes in the research proposal were approved by our funders, the NHS Executive South and West, in March 1998.

At this stage, we decided to take examples, as we found them, from the whole assessment spectrum – carers' needs assessments, carer involvement with an assessment and service reviews (IPPs) – asking professionals to pass on information about the project to any family where the carer's needs had been taken into account during the course of an assessment of a person with learning disabilities. In the case of children, this was quite often an ongoing process, rather than a discrete event. We also contacted day centres and asked the staff to pass on information about the study to families where the relative with a learning disability had recently had a service review (IPP).

In addition, as originally planned, quantitative data was collected in each area on the number and characteristics of carers who had received a formal carer's needs assessment or other forms of assessment. Carers' experiences could then be compared across different kinds of assessment process.

Revision to analysis of data

When we changed the research proposal, we also decided to tape record all the interviews, so that we could carry out a more detailed content analysis of the data. This enabled us to highlight the processes involved in assessments, and the reasons why they are effective or otherwise in different circumstances.

The original aim was to have 20 families in each authority. However, given the change in the proposal, we considered it more realistic and meaningful to interview a smaller number. This enabled us to conduct in-depth interviews, which were not limited to the question schedule, and to tape record and transcribe interviews. The subsequent analysis was grounded in the data,

identifying themes and interconnections from the carers' own words, by means of a charting process. We were able to raise some of the important issues again, on follow-up visits a year later, in order to check on carers' views, and to explore their own understanding of the support they had received.

The quantitative data obtained (eg satisfaction levels with services received and with aspects of the assessment) were analysed by a three-way comparison between carers' interviews, and the data obtained from people with learning disabilities and assessors.

Return visits

We returned after about one year to the families whom we had interviewed. The general aim was to examine the outcomes of the assessment, which had been the subject of the first interview. This phase proved to be an extremely important addition to the project, since it highlighted the fact that a carer assessment is only as good as its outcomes. We were also able to explore ways of making progress in meeting the support needs of these carers.

In the follow-up interviews, we again conducted semi-structured conversations, and obtained tape recordings for 36 out of 43 interviews. We also asked specific questions about satisfaction with the assessment, and about outcomes of services that had been assessed as needed.

The analysis of the final phase was twofold. In the first instance, we handled the data in a qualitative way, by examining for themes and interconnections, and on this occasion the analysis was aided by a computer package (Winmax, 1998). However, we also had details on interview schedules concerning the offers of service provision that had arisen from the assessments, and these were analysed quantitatively. In this final phase, we did not re-interview all the people with learning disabilities, but only those for whom there had been major changes. This resulted in six interviews, which lent themselves to analysis as individual case studies, based again on the themes suggested by the interviewees themselves.

Appendix B: Number and type of assessments

We obtained details of records for one year (1 April 1997–31 March 1998) within each of the five authorities from which it appeared that 157 people with learning disabilities had had an assessment of their needs. Of these, 56% were males and 44% females. They spanned both children and adults with an age range of 12–83 years but by far the most common age group was young adults (17–30 years), accounting for 48% of all cases assessed.

The vast majority of these assessments were carried out under the NHS and Community Care Act. In all cases, the individuals had the support of a family carer who was eligible for a Carers Act assessment. The table below shows the number of client assessments that led to any kind of carer's needs assessment between 1 April 1997 and 31 March 1998.

Type of assessment	Number	%
Full carer assessment	35	22
Partial assessment	79	50
No carers assessment	43	28
Total	**157**	**100**

Note: Partial assessments included any direct reference to the carer on the client's care plan or assessment form.

The records were examined in order to see when *any* reference had been made to different aspects of the carer's life and current role. The figures presented in the following table indicate that many carers are not being asked about issues that are likely to impact on their situation or capacity for caring.

Topics covered in carers' needs assessments

Topics	% over five areas
Carer's health	29
Carer's work	9
Housing	10
Carer's aspirations	39
Ability to continue caring	26

The majority of these 'client' cases (75%) were still open by the time the records search was complete. In some instances, this was up to six months later, suggesting that people with learning difficulties are seen as a priority for longer-term support. This, of course, means there is some hope of carers having their needs met, albeit sometimes indirectly, by requesting services for their relative.